I0120314

QUANTUM HUMAN

Embarking Fearlessly into a
New Era of Consciousness

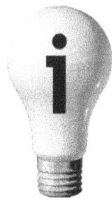

iBooks
Habent Sua Fata Libelli

Brian Clement, Ph.D., L.N.

iBooks
Manhanset House
Shelter Island Hts., New York 11965-0342

Tel: 212-427-7139

bricktower@aol.com • www.ibooksinc.com

All rights reserved under the International and Pan-American Copyright Conventions. No part of this publication may be reproduced, stored in a retrieval system, or transmitted in any form or by any means, electronic, or otherwise, without the prior written permission of the copyright holder. The iBooks colophon is a registered trademark of J. Boylston & Company, Publishers.

Library of Congress Cataloging-in-Publication Data
Clement, Brian B.

Quantum Human—Embarking Fearlessly Into A New Era Of Consciousness and Wellbeing
p. cm.

1. Health & Fitness—Homeopathy.

2. Health & Fitness—Naturopathy.

3. Health & Fitness—Longevity.

4. Biography & Autobiography—Science & Technology. Nonfiction, I. Title.

ISBN: 978-1-899694-32-2, Trade Paper • 978-1-899694-33-4, Hardcover

Copyright © 2025 by Brian R. Clement

May 2025

FOREWORD

Quantum Human, written by Dr. Brian Clement, is both a practical and visionary book. It's practical in the sense that it goes into the original researchers' work that was done to validate the teachings that are shared in this excellent offering.

It's visionary because he is able to go to the depths of these topics beyond just nutritional thinking. Quantum Human presents a vision of a total holistic way of life by increasing our bio frequency fields to their highest potential.

In this context, food is not simply calories but has important effects on our energy. Dr. Clement makes a very important point that can either raise our internal currents for superior health or lower our energy as a result of our lifestyle and diets, which leads to either radiant or poor outcomes. Our bio frequency determines how we communicate with the universe and with each other on more subtle cosmic planes.

He makes the visionary statement that we are all, in a sense, stardust interconnected by our frequencies to all of humanity and the multi universes. Quantum health has an exciting message of hope, possibility, and optimism that through the awareness of how to protect and build our energy, we can fulfill our total human potential.

As a part of his presentation, he brings in historical, cultural, and scientific sources to help us understand and validate our current knowledge of bio frequency and the potential applications for optimal health and well-being. In this process, he naturally shows the importance and necessity of transcending conventional scientific and allopathic belief systems, which currently have the status of "science."

In this process, he leads us to embrace a worldview that sees us as amplitude. Harmonics are connected to everything, and by improving these currents, we can experience the interconnection of all existence, helping us reach our optimal human potential.

He points out that deeper, authentic healing occurs when we build and repair those energy fields. And to this purpose, quantum healing includes the power of faith, positive placebo effect, gratitude, optimism, love, joy, helping other people, service, and charity, each of which have been proven to elevate wellbeing.

In contrast, he shows the negative health effects of nocebo, which has to do with how our negative thought forms will lead to illness.

He cites some powerful research and gives an interesting insight into live foods as a potent source of high-frequency bio photon energies that increase the body's pulse field. It was interesting to read his clinical research, which expresses that we can, within 18 days, actually begin to bring our energy to appropriate levels. He gives solid evidence that the live food cycle activates the interconnectedness of all existence. This is a beautiful, continual connection he makes in the offering.

I was particularly interested in the work with neuro-linguistics, which shows how the words we use affect our energy and communication to uplift the overall consciousness of ourselves, our communities, and literally of the planet. We must be energized.

He brings us a deeper understanding of the power of language and the energy characteristics in various communication systems that can really align us with the resonance of the universe. In conclusion, the understanding is that Brian has shown the transformative potential of subtle energy healing to help us move from what some people call anti-coherent patterns in their own field, and in our social field to create coherent patterns by showing us how to increase and harmonize our bioenergetic persona through the power of our thoughts and expressions.

In the conclusion of this book, Dr. Brian Clement introduces the exciting visionary idea of the Quantum Human State, which, as far as I understand via my half a century of work, is a really new concept. And he proves that this is the key to healing us individually and collectively in the 21st century. Quantum Human is about creating a total comprehensive lifestyle that leads us to raise our energy to its highest level in becoming a powerful human that can be physically, emotionally, mentally, and spiritually awake and effective.

This is an excellent practical and impactful book, not only for beginners but also for people who have been in this field of progressive health for years. It helps validate all the areas of work that advanced practitioners are doing and successfully brings the pieces together. I congratulate Clement for his excellent integration of all this information and for offering an outstanding way to think about building energy that gives us a deeper understanding of excellence and how to create it.

- Rabbi Gabriel Cousens, M.D., M.D. (Homeopathy), Doctor of Divinity, Diplomate in Ayurveda & Diplomate in Holistic Medicine

OVERVIEW

Quantum Humans
By Brian Clement, Ph.D., L.N.

Leaving the information age and rapidly moving into what I call "The age of consciousness" (AI) has the masses in a state of insecurity. *Quantum Human* is the remedy for you, to assure you that this time in history, humanity finally has a chance to get it right. There are endless examples and even more scientific research that shows modern biology, chemistry, and even genetics at some levels, have not gone far enough to uncover the inner workings of our human presence.

Unlike others who work exclusively in labs or on computer models, I have conducted clinical work for more than half a century, and the institute I direct pioneered the progressive health field 7 decades ago. We founded what is now called lifestyle medicine and applied this with hundreds of thousands of participants in our inhouse programs addressing longevity, disease, and wellbeing.

There is no doubt that what you will learn from this book is the future of medicine and healthcare. The only question is how long it will take for the ineffective, broken system to give way to noninvasive and powerfully productive processes that can remove many, if not all of the maladies, both psychological and physical, that the global population faces.

We invite you and all others to engage in your own life at such a level that you radiate confidence required to maintain youth, vitality, and strength. As self-healers with assertive independence there is nothing you cannot achieve.

Outlined in the pages of *Quantum Human* is the blueprint for you to partake of the new world and manifest whatever it is that your purest and heartfelt desires are.

As people living at a time where consciousness prevails with thorough knowledge of the workings of wisdom, there is no longer any excuse to limit your internal power. This gift is not one that makes you be feared but conversely respected for your level of commitment and integrity that all possess.

DEDICATION

To the late Dr. Hunt, who sat patiently with me and encouraged this literary project in her home overlooking the pacific. To Randall Fitzgerald, who worked tirelessly with research and editing. To my assistant Susan Maharaj, my son Blake Clement, and most of all, Iesha Beene, who endured hundreds of hours of exploration in writing – rewriting and never did anything but support and assist.

To all my fellow seekers and scientists who long for the soon-to-come day when we abolish the fragile framework of modern healthcare and reassemble the effective and noninvasive methods that are discussed in this book and the most important science laboratories conducting advanced projects globally.

YOU, THE READER, CAN EMPLOY THIS FRAMEWORK TO ERRADICATE, PREVENT, AND STOP PREMATURE AGING AND DISEASE AND THE ONSETTLED LIFE THAT FOSTERS THEIR CREATION.

ADDITIONAL SOURCES ON THE SUBJECT

Cell biologist Bruce Lipton's book, *The Biology of Belief: Unleashing the Power of Consciousness (Hay House, 2005, ISBN: 9781401923440)*, a consciousness-based understanding of human biology, has been a worldwide success over the past decade; by comparison, *Quantum Human* updates, expands and makes current the state of science in the field of mind/body medicine.

Other big-sellers that touch on themes in *Quantum Human* include:

Molecules of Emotion: The Science Behind Mind-Body Medicine, by Candace Pert, Ph.D. *(Simon & Schuster, 1999, ISBN: 9780684846347)*. How our thoughts and emotions affect our health, based on the chemical network inside our bodies linking thoughts and cellular activities.

You Are the Placebo: Making Your Mind Matter, by Dr. Joe Dispenza (Hay House, 2015, *ISBN: 978-1401944582*). How is it possible to heal the body by thought alone? (In less than six months since its publication, this book received more than 650 reader reviews on Amazon; it has also become a New York Times bestseller.)

I DO NOT CONDONE ANIMAL SUFFERING IN SCIENCE.

CHAPTER SUMMARIES

Chapter 1: Bio-Frequency Medicine

This chapter introduces the concept of bio-frequency medicine, focusing on how universal rhythms and bio-energy fields influence health. It explains how subtle energy particles, which balance protons, neutrons, atoms, and molecules, form the foundation of life. Imbalances in these particles can lead to disease, and bio-frequency therapies are presented as a means of restoring balance and healing.

Chapter 2: History of Energy as a Tool

This chapter explores the history of how energy has been used as a tool for healing and human advancement. It looks at ancient cultures' understanding of bio-energy fields, from using natural energy vortexes for building sites to the early 20th-century discoveries in quantum physics. The chapter emphasizes that modern science is now rediscovering the interconnectedness of energy and healing.

Chapter 3: Anatomy of a 'Miracle'

This chapter explores spontaneous remission of cancer and other radical healings that seem like "miracles." It examines the story of Mitchell May, who survived a devastating car accident. His recovery was marked by what doctors deemed miraculous regeneration, leading to the avoidance of a leg amputation. The chapter highlights how the power of belief and the human biofield can influence such unexpected healing.

Chapter 4: An Energy Affecting Humans and Animals

Experiments at Indiana University School of Medicine showed that lab animals, such as cancer-infected mice, experienced remission after energy healing sessions. This chapter discusses how the exchange of biofield energy—through focused intention and care—can affect both humans and animals. The experiments raise important questions about how bio-energy can potentially impact human diseases like cancer.

Chapter 5: Reaffirming Ancient Healing Principles

This chapter traces the history of healing through energy, from ancient practices like 'laying-on-of-hands' to modern scientific validation of these methods. Historical figures like Hippocrates and Benjamin Franklin studied such healing principles, leading to modern explorations of energy's influence on the body. The chapter discusses how ancient techniques are still relevant today.

Chapter 6: Science Validates the Human Energy Field

Research from UCLA and Yale validates that humans are bioelectric beings emitting bio-frequency energies. This chapter examines how ancient healing practices like Qi Gong and acupuncture manipulate these fields. It also highlights studies showing that animals and fish, such as deep-sea creatures, emit bio-electric signals that can be measured scientifically.

Chapter 7: We Are All 'Light' Beings

Scientists in Japan first discovered that humans emit biophotons (light) from their bodies. This chapter explains how biophoton emissions are linked to health, noting that healthier individuals emit stronger light. Meditation is shown to boost biophoton emissions, and healers who practice meditation can transfer this light to others, enhancing the healing process.

Chapter 8: Light Treatment Gains Acceptance

Light therapy has gained recognition for treating various health conditions, including chronic fatigue and Alzheimer's disease. This chapter explores how ancient wisdom about light's healing properties is now being scientifically validated, with different wavelengths of light proving to have profound therapeutic effects.

Chapter 9: The Healing Power of Subtle Energy Medicine

The work of Dr. Valerie Hunt at UCLA is highlighted, focusing on how diseases stem from anti-coherent patterns in human bio-energy fields. The chapter explores how energy devices can diagnose illnesses before symptoms appear and how human intention and bio-energy healing, such as Edd Edwards' directed energy techniques, have measurable effects on human health.

Chapter 10: Nourish Your Cells, Replenish Your Energy Field

This chapter emphasizes the importance of living, organic foods for replenishing the human energy field. It discusses how synthetic and processed foods drain this bio-energy, while raw foods like kale and wheatgrass contain micro-currents that boost the immune system and promote health.

Chapter 11: Thoughts Channel Healing Energy

Thoughts and beliefs are shown to channel healing energy through consciousness. The chapter discusses how stress reduction, meditation, and prayer can alter cellular-level processes and enhance healing. It explores the placebo effect and how our mindset and thoughts can be powerful tools for self-healing.

Chapter 12: Three Healing 'Vibes': Loving Kindness, Forgiveness, and Gratitude

Emotions like love, kindness, forgiveness, and gratitude are described as bio-electromagnetic frequencies that can positively impact health. This chapter explores the scientific data supporting how these emotions influence healing, countering the damaging effects of chronic stress and anger on the bio-electric system.

Chapter 13: Practices and Technologies for Bio-frequency Healing

Various technologies, such as biofeedback, hypnosis, visualization, and meditation, are discussed in this chapter, showing how they manipulate the biofield to promote healing. The chapter also explores the ancient practice of acupuncture and how it aligns with modern energy therapies like the Emotional Freedom Technique (EFT).

Chapter 14: Your Frequency Vibrates Universal Energy

This chapter discusses how human frequency connects with the universal energy that governs all life. The chapter suggests that healing is proportionate to one's openness and consciousness, and it delves into how individuals can access and harness this energy for self-healing.

Chapter 15: Quantum Living

The final chapter ties together the concepts from the previous chapters, emphasizing the limitless potential of humans as quantum beings. It discusses how living in alignment with bio-frequency principles and energy awareness can lead to healthier, more harmonious lives, both individually and collectively.

TABLE OF CONTENTS

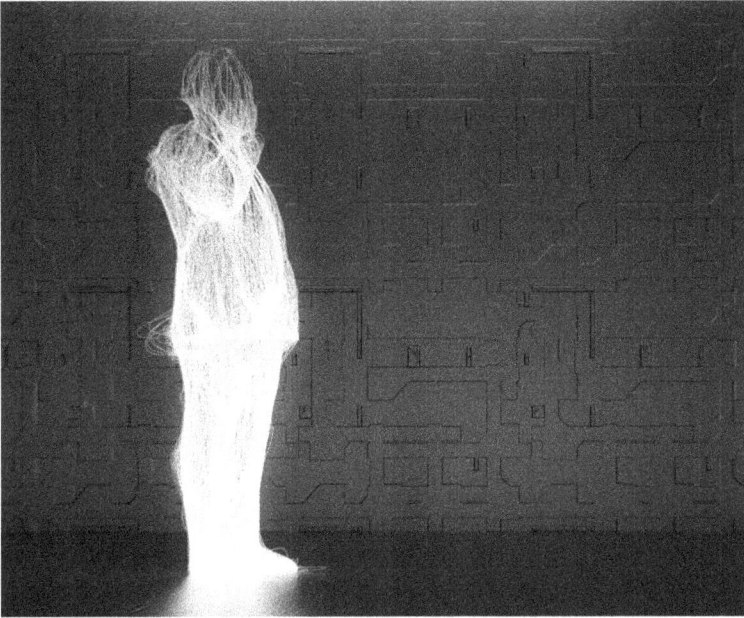

INTRODUCTION:

Sparking like a bolt of lightning, a synaptic nerve firing, or the glint in a lover's eyes, each one of us was brought into this world through a cataclysmic event. In 2016, researchers at Northwestern University captured something extraordinary as they peered through the lenses of their microscopes. At the instant a sperm fertilizes an egg, billions of zinc ions are released in a radiant cascade of energy, illuminating the conception of life itself. This flash of light is more than just a scientific marvel—it is a profound symbol of creation. It signifies the creative force that defines humanity and separates us from the artificial. The brilliance of this spark casts light in all directions allowing us to see more clearly our essence. It invites us to explore a deeper truth: that life, at its core, is an intricate interplay of energy, biology, and potential. And it is precisely that potential wherein life steps into the quantum realm. This is the starting point of our journey into the mysteries of existence, where science and wonder converge to redefine what it means to be alive.

This book, Quantum Human, explores how we are connected to the quantum physics that underlies our reality. It bridges the gap between quantum mechanics and biology, uncovering how our physical, mental, and spiritual existence is deeply intertwined with the fundamental principles of the universe. From groundbreaking experiments to the theoretical foundations laid by pioneers like Max Planck, Albert Einstein, and Erwin Schrödinger, we will journey into the frontier where quantum mechanics and biology converge. Together, we will explore the profound implications of these discoveries for healthcare, human potential, and our collective future.

For centuries, ancient traditions and practices like meditation, acupuncture, and energy healing reflected an intuitive understanding of the subtle forces that govern life. These methods, rooted in the belief that unseen energies influence health and harmony, were once dismissed as pseudoscience by the modern world. However, as scientific advancements uncover the quantum principles that underpin cellular processes, consciousness, and the very fabric of existence, these ancient approaches are being reevaluated. What was once regarded as superstition now finds validation in research showing how quantum mechanics shapes the interconnected systems that sustain life, bridging the gap between ancient wisdom and modern science.

Quantum Human delves into this interplay between ancient practices and cutting-edge science. By examining concepts like bio-energy, quantum consciousness, and the quantum mechanisms driving our biology, this book challenges readers to expand their perception of reality. We are not merely products of genetics and environment; we are beings woven into the quantum fabric of the universe, with creative potential as limitless as the cosmos itself.

We find ourselves in a transformative era where old axioms are dissolving, and science reveals ever-deeper layers of reality. Quantum mechanics allows us to peer into the essence of life, while emerging technologies like artificial intelligence and virtual reality immerse us in experiences that challenge our understanding of what it means to be human. Yet, as we embrace this age of artifice, it is crucial to remember the unique spark of creation that defines us—not just at conception but in every thought, action, and impulse. This quantum essence, boundless and creative, is what separates humanity from its artificial creations.

By understanding our quantum nature, we can move toward a future where humanity thrives—not by mimicking machines, but by unlocking the potential within ourselves. Imagine a world where boundaries dissolve, and individuals work in harmony, supported by a deep understanding of their interconnectedness. This vision is not speculative—it is within reach. By harnessing the principles of quantum physics, we can expand our awareness, develop untapped abilities, and redefine what it means to flourish as human beings.

In Quantum Human, you are invited to embark on a journey that blends scientific rigor, philosophical reflection, and practical application. Together, we will uncover how quantum knowledge can illuminate a path forward—one where health, consciousness, and harmony flourish.

The story of quantum biology begins at the dawn of the 20th century, when classical physics—the cornerstone of our understanding of the natural world—faced a profound crisis. Scientists studying how heated objects emit light found that existing theories predicted an impossible result: as the frequency of light increased, the energy emitted should skyrocket to infinity. This bizarre and nonsensical outcome, known as the "ultraviolet catastrophe," completely contradicted experimental observations, which showed that energy emission actually tapered off at higher frequencies. This glaring mismatch between theory and reality revealed that the traditional laws of physics were insufficient to explain how energy behaved at very small scales. Faced with this conundrum, physicists were forced to rethink the very nature of energy itself. In 1900, Max Planck proposed a groundbreaking idea: energy isn't continuous but comes in tiny, discrete packets he called quanta. This discovery laid the foundation for quantum mechanics, a science that revealed the world at its smallest scales operates in strange and surprising ways. For life, this insight was monumental. It suggested that processes we take for granted—like how plants convert sunlight into energy or how molecules interact in our bodies—are governed by these quantum rules. Planck's discovery not only saved physics but opened the door to understanding life at its most fundamental level.

Shortly afterward, Albert Einstein expanded on Planck's work by studying light. Classical physics viewed light as a wave, but Einstein proposed that light also behaves as tiny particles, called photons, not unlike Planck's quanta. These photons, he explained, could strike a material and knock out electrons—a phenomenon known as the photoelectric effect. This discovery not only won Einstein a Nobel Prize but also helped reveal light's dual nature—it can behave as both a wave and a particle depending on how we observe it. And more importantly, this laid the foundation for a new understanding of how light powers life. Photons power the process of photosynthesis, through which all plants convert sunlight into energy to sustain themselves—and ultimately, the entire food chain.

As quantum mechanics evolved, scientists began to ask: could quantum principles apply to matter itself, not just energy like light? In 1924, Louis de Broglie made a stunning claim: everything in the universe, from electrons to entire atoms, behaves both like particles (tiny bits of matter) and waves (spread-out energy patterns). Picture throwing a pebble into a pond: you'd see ripples spreading outward like waves. De Broglie showed that even the pebble itself—on a quantum scale—has wave-like properties. This concept, called wave-particle duality, blurred the lines between physics and biology, raising intriguing questions about how quantum principles might govern life.

One of the most significant breakthroughs came from Erwin Schrödinger, who used de Broglie's ideas to create the wave equation. This equation doesn't tell us exactly where a particle is, but rather the probabilities of where it might be—introducing the idea that, at the quantum level, nothing is certain. Schrödinger later explored the connection between quantum mechanics and life in his book What is Life?. He suggested that quantum principles might explain how DNA stays stable and how genetic information is transferred with such precision, laying the groundwork for a new field: quantum biology.

Around the same time, Werner Heisenberg introduced the Uncertainty Principle, which states that we can never know both a particle's exact position and momentum at the same time. It's like trying to measure a bird in flight—you can either track where it is or how fast it's going, but not both. This uncertainty, once thought to apply only to subatomic particles, turned out to have profound biological implications. For example, it plays a role in enzymatic reactions, where molecules interact with astonishing speed and precision, seemingly guided by quantum rules.

As quantum mechanics developed, scientists began to connect these principles to specific biological processes. By the mid-20th century, Pascual Jordan proposed that quantum effects might influence large-scale biological phenomena like photosynthesis and vision. For example, in photosynthesis, quantum principles such as coherence allow plants to transport energy with near-perfect efficiency. This means energy can move through molecules like a well-coordinated relay team, without any getting lost along the way—something classical physics struggles to explain.

More recently, Jim Al-Khalili and Johnjoe McFadden at the University of Surrey explain how quantum tunneling—a phenomenon where particles pass through energy barriers that should be impassable—may play a crucial role in biology. For instance, tunneling helps explain how enzymes accelerate chemical reactions, ensuring they happen fast enough to sustain life. Similarly, quantum mechanics may explain how our sense of smell works. When we detect a scent, tiny particles in our nose may "vibrate" in ways that rely on quantum principles, allowing us to distinguish between different scent molecules.

The story of quantum physics reaches its most profound culmination in the exploration of quantum human biology, where the mysteries of consciousness and the essence of what makes us uniquely human come into focus. Researchers like Valerie Hunt at the University of California, Los Angeles have explored how quantum interactions might govern bio-energy fields, suggesting that our bodies generate energy flows that influence health and healing. This idea, once dismissed as pseudoscience, is gaining traction as we uncover more about how energy fields interact with cells and tissues. Meanwhile, Nobel Laureate Roger Penrose and anesthesiologist Stuart Hameroff proposed that quantum coherence—the ability of particles to remain interconnected over distance—might influence consciousness itself.

Today, quantum biology is uncovering the hidden quantum forces that shape some of the most essential processes in living organisms.

From the near-perfect efficiency of photosynthesis to the precision of enzymatic reactions and the potential role of quantum effects in brain function, this field reveals that life operates at the edge of two worlds: the quantum and the classical. Far from being mere chemical randomness, life emerges as an intricate, ordered system deeply connected to the quantum fabric of reality.

At its core, quantum biology shows us that life is more than a series of chemical reactions—it is a precise, elegant interplay of particles, waves, and energy. These discoveries are not just advancing our understanding of biological processes; they are challenging our perception of existence itself. What is life? What sustains it? And how does humanity—with its unique creativity and consciousness—fit into this vast quantum tapestry? By delving into these questions, quantum biology opens a doorway to reimagining not only what it means to be alive but also the extraordinary potential we hold within.

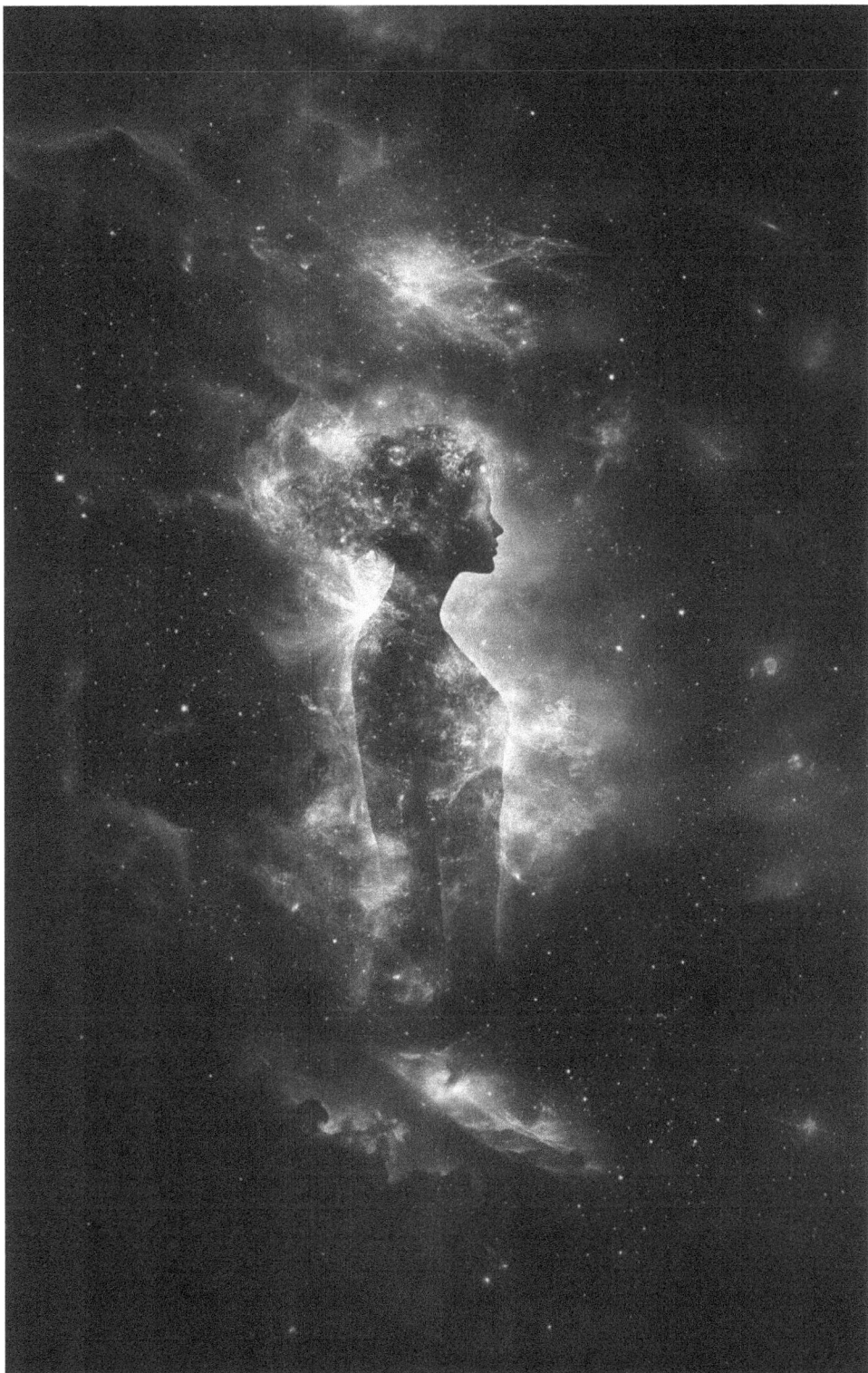

CHAPTER 1:

Bio-Frequency Medicine

"Your ability to hear me now is because there are cells in your ears that are converting sound waves into an electrical signal, which is what the brain can interpret as acoustics," - Francis Ashcroft (Royal Society GlaxoSmithKline Research Professor at the University Laboratory of Physiology, Oxford, and a Fellow of Trinity College, Oxford.)

Have you been feeling confused about the future and what it may bring? Our health, the planet we reside on, and the abundant instability worldwide render a sense of unease. Institutions that we have been reliant on are crumbling and are often corrupt at the core. What is it then that we can trust? Maybe the answer is simpler than we realize. Universal rhythms that govern all biology and chemistry work with utter perfection and balance. By submitting ourselves to deeply studying and thoroughly comprehending this pinnacle system of perfection and mimicking it, we, for the first time, can tap into the power and splendor of health, happiness, and healing.

Space, time, energy, and matter began the birthing process between 13 and 14 billion years ago.[15] Approximately 3 and a half billion years ago, special molecules combined to form large intricate structures called matter, which then coalesced into what we call organisms and materialized approximately two and a half billion years later. Our ancestors, in their original form, arrived approximately 100,000 – 200,000 years ago; this was the start of the voyage that we historically call human life. From the endless expanse of darkness, existence seeded itself and grew into everything that we have ever known.[16]

Deep Dive

Over the last half-century, I have witnessed the precipitous growth of Western medical ideologies and their repercussions. Even well-meaning progressive scientists cage their protocols by systematizing a scientific process. Apparently, the conventional perception of what matters is limited to the veneer or surface of any given pursuit. We look at cells but fail to ask the question, "What creates these remarkable lifeforms?" In sketching out the anatomy, we may hypothesize and then unquestionably establish how these cells, which create skeletal structures and organs, biochemically function. When it comes to the brain and the mind it houses, we are even less able to agree on its significant role in biological health. For these reasons, I have focused my efforts on natural history, both Newtonian and Quantum physics, chemistry, biology, and other advanced sciences. In this inaugural chapter, I will describe how I believe all life is manifested, created, and catapulted into existence. There is a logical pattern that emerges when we begin to appreciate the multitude of factors that exist in our current understanding of the full spectrum of science.

By evaluating thousands of participants in the Hippocrates Health Institute programs, with elaborate blood profiles, bio-frequency interpretations of organ systems, and functional assessments of potential disease states and/or disease I have accrued knowledge on the universal systems that govern physical health. More important is a mounting arsenal of technological therapies that reach deeply into the physical realm and help to adjust the resonating forces that manifest tissue. Clinically observing the results of such treatment has led to a body of evidence that cannot be refuted. This field of *HUMAN QUANTUM BIOLOGY* was pioneered long before the applications that I speak of were available.

When literally tracing the origins of life, you can clearly see that the most subtle particles are the core of all organisms. When these particles are working with the balance between protons, neutrons, atoms, and molecules, there is a homeostasis that reigns. By throwing off even one of these particles, imbalance follows, and if unchecked, can manifest into disease. This offering will lay out a concise archetype that can be employed in your life. There are many categories and realms to review in this quest. As you will learn, there is a multitude of procedures and treatments that can be useful in healing. Gathering a chorus of correct bio-frequency therapies combined with a lifestyle that is amenable to universal resonance will ensure your progress toward equilibrium.

Unified Thought

There are new challenges to the "Big Bang" theory of our universe's conception. The very idea of a single universe has long since been disproven. Recent findings conclude that there are many, likely infinite, numbers of universes.[17] When the Mars probe penetrated deep space, it sent back data and photographs revealing new findings that reestablished the former hypotheses that discussed the expansiveness of an endless existence. One way for you to understand this reality is if you picture a large flattened circle (dark hole) that has two lines protruding downward from the 3 and 9 o'clock positions defining the cone shape, then somewhere in the middle, the lines start to return creating the mirror image and ending at another flattened circle.

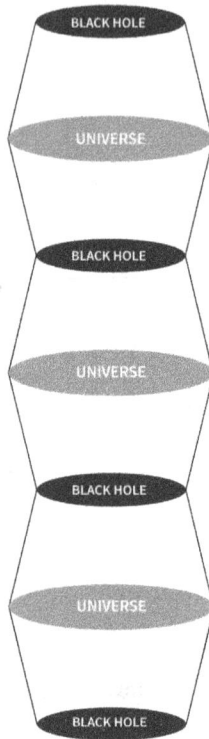

These dark holes are actually portholes connecting universes. Residing between each of these conduits, there is a universe unto itself with unique terrestrial life. This life is generated by the particular planets and stars within this cone (universe). Like the cosmos we reside in, stars, planets, galaxies, and their cyclical motions interact, creating a celestial system perpetuating its own energetic and gravitational cycle. We now believe that highly charged particles can move from one universe to the other, creating a continuum of perpetual connectivity. Today's astronomy and space science, with its advanced technologies, are unlocking what were previously mysteries or theories only considered by the most avant-garde thinkers.

In 1898, Max Planck and many of his colleagues began delving into what is now known as Particle Theory or Quantum Mechanics. Max Planck, the early 20th century premier physicist, published a landmark paper called "Zur Theorie des Gesetzes der Energieverteilung im

Normalspektrum" (On the Theory of the Law of Energy Distribution in the Normal Spectrum) galvanizing the Quantum Theory[18].

Planck's work was published in the *Annalen der Physik*. His work is summarized in two books *Thermodynamik* (Thermodynamics) (1897) and *Theorie der Wärmestrahlung* (Theory of heat radiation) (1906). These early quantum physicists were aided by Einstein with his theory of relativity. Pondering the endless expanse, well beyond protons and neutrons, he stated that all life is born of minute frequencies. Even Einstein's' hypotheses have been surpassed, which he predicted would happen more than a century ago.[19] Minute particles that are born out of frequencies have established the entirety of what we consider reality, both on a physical and conceptual level. The very energetic stars that are integral to the function of our and any other universe are the manifestations of the exact particles and frequencies that present physical form.

In our specific solar system, the universe generates life from the star we call the sun. It is 98% light gases (74% Hydrogen, 24% Helium) and only 2% heavier elements like oxygen, carbon, neon, iron, and others.[20] These elements are often referred to as "metals" in astronomical terms, even though they include non-metallic elements like oxygen. In the center of the sun, every second, infinite amount of protons are generated. They instantly begin colliding with neutrons, creating friction and heat. This process continues for approximately 100,000 years as new protons continue to push forward. Upon reaching the outer edges of the sun, a solar storm or flair often occurs when magnetic energy stored in the Sun's atmosphere is suddenly released. This dynamically ejects photons in the form of light and other types of electromagnetic radiation.

Similarly, it also releases a stream of charged particles (mostly protons and electrons) called Solar Energetic Particles (SEPs). When a solar flare occurs, it can accelerate these particles to very high energies into space. When these particles interact with other particles or magnetic fields, they immediately lose energy in the form of photons.[21] This light is moving so rapidly it only requires 8 ½ minutes to reach earth, where it is captured in great part by green leafy plants. The seasons are molded by this process, as well as the sun's proximity to the earth we all inhabit. Today's advanced discoveries have shown that life in kind is generated by light, resulting in everything that we consider matter actually being particles of frequencies that have gathered together. These particles copulate into a multitude of unique forms. Some are trees, some are birds, and others humans. The periodic table, which contains 118 known elements, is all part of the sun's gasses.

Periodic Table of Elements

Astronomers who have studied the composition of the sun have cataloged 67 chemical elements in the star. There may be more but in amounts too small for instruments to detect.

Here is a table of the 10 most common elements in the sun:

Element	Abundance (pct. of total number of atoms)	Abundance (pct. of total mass)
Hydrogen	91.2	71.0
Helium	8.7	27.1
Oxygen	0.078	0.97
Carbon	0.043	0.40
Nitrogen	0.0088	0.096
Silicon	0.0045	0.099
Magnesium	0.0038	0.076

Credits: Space.com [22]

Each of these elements is literally part of all lifeforms, including our own bodies. This living earth we inhabit harbors in its core the ancient photonic energies previously projected from the sun. These energies magnetically interact with the cosmos, manifesting the polar movement of the earth, the currents of the ocean, and the blood flowing in our veins.

Since we now know that stardust's energetic particles create structure, it should not be a stretch for us to recognize that properly arranged assemblages of these ions render health and well-being. Unfortunately, disorganized frequency, be it planetary or man-made, disrupts homeostasis often causing physical disorder. As one example, high levels of disrupted photons collected in one defined area can actually mutate cells, causing tumor growth, among other maladies. Dr. Devra Davis exposed the radiation hazard from electronic devices, like cell phones and tablets.[23] This demonstrates how today's electronic age has precipitated a new challenge, creating unique disease states due to exposure to renegade frequencies. Cellular systems that were born out of the Pentagon's arsenal have been reliant upon Wi-Fi technology, a frequency that mimics water. The next step, which is called Li-Fi (5G), mirrors the frequency of oxygen. This is concerning as the further we move away from the healthy established structural systems and begin to manipulate the very sources of life, like water and oxygen, the more we pervade the biological systems that we must protect to preserve future life. There is great public concern about the effects of 5G technologies and their effects on the molecular structure of oxygen and its absorption by human beings and other creatures.

Inversely, when mimicking the origins of the multiple universes and the dark holes that create zero-point gravity, we can actually help to heal and reverse maladies. Two harmonious frequencies have been used throughout history that are born out of sound frequencies. One is 424, and the other is 528; each of them has therapeutic effects on your well-being, both biological and psychological. The latter helps to calm the systems; the first helps you to focus. There are many more attributes, but these are the core benefits.

Think of zero-point gravity as the quietest space in existence. This state of virtual nothingness is the birthplace of protons, neutrons, atoms, molecules, and matter (structure). The conventional scientist or mathematician may ask, how does nothing create something? For Quantum biologists it is this profoundly exhilarating perspective that can provide the pathway to creating either physical well-being or disastrous disorder. In this book, I will present scientific studies that confirm how we internally work via bio-frequencies and how these particles connect us to all other life on this planet, in our universe, and beyond our confined planetary system. Shattering conventional limitations will provide future scientists the wisdom to conquer even the greatest diseases once and for all. We can harmonize with our environment and prevent the unnecessary problems that are created when we ignore the state of our epigenetics. Epigenetics is defined as the study of gene expression which causes change in organisms because of the modification of genes rather than the alteration of the genetic code itself. What this means is that everything from our thoughts to our environment can instantly affect our genome. As an example, your gut has two hundred times the genes than the rest of your body. This is the science to support the significance of both immune and affirmative mental patterns since 80% of the cells of the immune system are trained and regulated due to the presence of healthy bacteria in the gut[24]. Imagine the proper utilization of pro-body frequencies in correcting disorders. This is the new frontier of human health care.

Many indigenous tribes inherently knew that healing was achieved when using all the forces of nature. Many spoke of fire and water, others of symbolic creatures, astronomy, and esoteric spirituality. Today, progressive science is validating traditional methods as viable tools in the conquest of disease.[25] As we marry these aboriginal practices with bio-frequency medicine, we will once again tap into the origins of creation and manifest healing with ease.

Reality or Consciousness or Both?

Liberating our minds from the rigid confines of established thinking and academic standards is difficult. One must be willing to ask the deeper questions of what exists beyond the currently accepted dogma. As an example, you may meet a brilliant computer programmer, and when asking her how the technology works, she may not know at all. Life is often placed on automatic pilot whereas we are performing spectacular activities without fully grasping what it takes to achieve these feats. Currently, science is looking at the facade rather than asking how the facade was created.

Future science and the pioneers in the conquest of abolishing status quo standards have now presented hybrid intelligence biometric avatars (HIBA)[26]. Philosophers for millennia have discussed unified consciousness, but today, it is a real process that technology brings us. There will be a rapidly ever-increasing accessible database of infinite knowledge that can afford each of us greater insight and wisdom since it will have the ability to collect data itself and ask questions verbally.

It will be able to think in a way that is truly outside the box as its thought process would be something completely different from what any human has done before.

Ultimately, when the masses individually access this, there will be a common universal consciousness that emerges. This means that many of the perplexing problems that our species has endured from the dawn of time will be resolved since our critical consciousness will be able to dissect the causative reasons for problematic concerns and simultaneously find a resolution that everyone will agree upon. Imagine what the future holds when everything from disease to poverty to war is no longer part of our future.

One of my phobias is driving over bridges, namely the Golden Gate in San Francisco and the George Washington in New York City. For some reason, as I navigate these roadways, I think of the Godzilla movies where the monster reached up and sent these strong suspended structures crumbling into the water. Somehow, each year, I find myself driving over these frightening, engineered marvels. However, my mind is always, paradoxically, at ease since I know that the strong steel that holds these landmarks together has been holding these bridges up for multiple decades. My fears remain high in light of quantum theory, though. Knowing that even the strongest metals have less than 2% structure and approximately 98% the absence of structure causes me apprehension. Considering such insight, is a bridge perception or reality?

Advanced scientists often use unconventional tools to unravel complicated problems. One of these tools that is commonly employed is light and energy measuring photography. This Petrographic Microscope, using a specialized chromium film procedure, measures bio-energy fields of living plants and human anatomy by viewing the Chondrule crystal composition and quantity. This is one technology employed in quantum measurement. When removing a section of a leaf, we have obviously discarded some of the matter-based structure. Yet, this particular photographic technique reveals the energetic outline of the part of the leaf that was discarded.

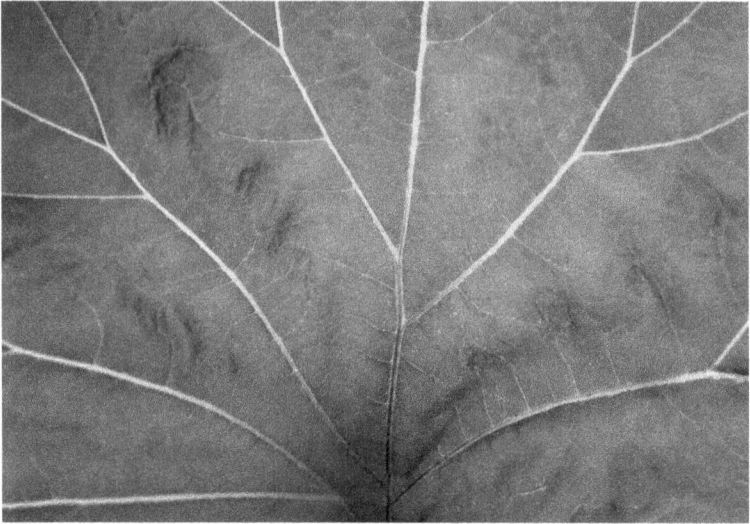

In the past, this would have been called esoteric and mystical; today, it is called Quantum Biology. Throughout this book, I will present evidence of this emerging science and many of the courageous pioneers who have been willing to stake their professional careers, challenging the standard. We can no longer allow the forces that manipulate and control our culture to dominate our academic and personal lives. Unlocking the genius of how all life works will bring us knowledge and tools to create unified harmony in our health and world. We all know that a one-inch move in the right or wrong direction can create a lifesaving event or imminent demise. We are at the cusp of the revolution, where progressive humanity will take the reins and lead us into a new sphere of positive influence. Thus, we must be uncompromising and vigorous in our pursuit.

Light, in its natural state, harmoniously permeates our environment. If we manipulate a laser (light) to a focused point, it can cut through steel. One analogy that highlights how frequencies govern all that exists is the way the keystone instrument, the piano, resonates sound via frequencies. Conversely, discord emanates whenever the strings are slightly loosened. Notes can become noise when they do not resonate in the atmosphere that surrounds us. This helps us to understand how emerging light particle technologies in the conquest of disease and suffering are the future of medicine.

Hippocrates Health Institute, which I have had the privilege to direct, along with my wife, Anna Maria, since 1980, has significantly employed energy field technology in the lifestyle protocols that we teach each of our participants. As science dramatically expands its depth of technological quantum knowledge, each generation of these tools is increasingly employed in assisting those with a wide variety of disorders. For decades, we have clinically observed the impressive difference in health improvements via testing. Our medical team employs a plethora of bio-chemical and bio-frequency methods and technologies in assisting the people we work with so that their immune system exponentially advances, aiding recovery. Knowing that the cell is a combination of biochemistry and biological frequency, we are completely committed to fully supporting the maximum function attainable.

We aspire to achieve full knowledge and implementation of light frequencies and electromagnetic pulsations in the conquest of reversing biological disorder. At the same time, we cannot forget that our role is that of facilitators, not manipulators. Figuratively, our task is to discover the specific musical note which is the basis of all life. At this very moment, progressive science is in the process of tuning the instrument and coming closer to the perfect resonance for healing. Historically, medicine has dissected, dismembered, and altered biological order in hopes of composing the perfect symphony. However, the proper instruments already exist in our natural world. We simply have to hit the right notes. Is it not more effective to learn how the universe functions rather than trying to stop its inherent unfolding? Mainstream scientists believe that the proper course to take is aggressive intervention, whereas Quantum science supports respectful, subtle changes fostering successful outcomes. The current methods have systemically failed when it comes to delivering universally positive results. As Johns Hopkins Medical Institute reports, "standard protocols and pharmaceutical usage has risen to one of the most formidable killers in developed societies today; this is the 3rd leading cause of death in the US." If this is not enough to provoke change, then I don't know what is. At present, the consequences of our systematic approaches appear unchangeable. We must apply the brake, come to our rational senses, and work in harmony with the natural world rather than disregarding it. Medical models are necessary, yet should be encouraged to constantly improve and change.

Our professional mission as healthcare practitioners is to constantly tweak and advance our current methods while remaining open to new data from good science. Somehow, our relentless pursuit of achieving excellence has left the excellence part out, preventing us from learning and growing. Professional careers are often built on faulty, antiquated information.

Ridiculed are the pioneers who break the patterns and challenge the standard dogma. Ultimately, TRUTH reigns, creating levity that governs good decisions. This eventually results in the masses relinquishing their learned rigidity. Throughout history, we have seen that pioneers who spark leaps of consciousness always liberate us to move closer to our "better" selves.

- The Wright brothers were mocked for their 'outrageous' attempts to fly.

- Aristotle spoke of self-governance and led his students to become totally responsible for themselves, though, at the time, this was considered heresy. We now model democratic governments from his contributions.

- Dr. Martin Luther King expressed that love is more powerful than hate, and he was able to turn the tide of suffering for multitudes of people who had previously been oppressed and suppressed by compassionless authoritarians.

Science is now poised to make a decision. Will we surge forward to assist a suffering and broken humanity, or will we err on the side of conventional institutions and remain a shadow of our greatness?

Quantum Human will bring you stories, data, scientifically proven technologies, and pertinent history that will liberate the open-minded reader to be in awe of the future and its emerging medicine. Only you can affirm your acceptance of unlimited potential by rising to the steadfast position that is now required. My view is that we have seen the 'light,' and that is what we should all be focused on. Reasonable women and men who desire concrete progress have always opened the way to greatness by shedding previous notions that often failed us.

New science will embrace amplified imagination so that restrictive thoughts do not impair the potential to discover excellence. Scientists should be proud and brave enough to leave behind the comfortable confines of institutionalized practice. Not long ago, a surgeon would have scoffed at laser or robotic surgery, but now they are considered commonplace. In the next generation of pioneering physicists, biologists, and chemists, we will break through the thin veil between current practice and innovative success. As an example, most academics would deny the proven fact that light and sound waves actually permeate and move through thick metal walls, coming out and continuing intact on the other side. Since this has been filmed, I do not think it is wise to denounce this newly discovered reality.

Recent studies revealed that the father's lifestyle might influence fetal development long before the sperm are en route to meet the egg, precipitating personality, and genetic traits in the soon-to-come embryo. Formerly, we believed that the anatomy and psychology of the host father were purely from the DNA traits developed over many generations. This new finding acknowledges that direct intervention from today's epigenetics (lifestyle)influences the baby as much, if not more so, as the classic gene theory.[27][28][29]

Rather than fighting the tide of exciting progress, we should be elated that the heavy burden of holding up antiquated ideas can be dismissed. Each of you reading this book must discuss it with people of influence. You can gently challenge their ideas by proposing that they see things in a different way, hoping this will bring about change.

My objective is to present a wide range of advanced knowledge on the subject of energy as a healer. We will begin in the upcoming chapters by explaining the phenomenon of human-to-human touch therapy. This organic yet scientifically proven method has consistently been shown to enhance health and healing. You will be introduced to many pioneering giants in the field of advanced bio-frequency medicine so that you can learn of the brilliant and outstanding work that has brought us to our current plateau of validity in this emerging field. From our thoughts to man-made technology that projects positive healing frequencies to the negative electrical currents that emanate from modern devices, we are all swimming in a soup of bio-frequency fields. Your biggest leap will be to accept yourself as light particles rather than the individual who looks back at you from the mirror. Our stoic, concrete persona seems quite important, yet is actually more fragile than the frequencies that are in constant flux creating your cells, including your skeletal structure and organs.

I'll present state-of-the-art knowledge and science on this subject but do not be fooled into thinking that there is no more work to be done. At this moment, I believe in the necessity of laying the new rails down so that the high-speed train that is being assembled will have an exceedingly refined route to elevate biology and science into an enlightened, non-invasive realm. Cumulatively, advanced thinkers should bridge the divide and together imagine and build a finer future. There is no longer time for ego or arrogance. We must humble ourselves and relegate discord to the history books. Viewing the future positively will reward us in unfathomable ways. As you move forward in your own life, access the abundant tools of light, sound, energy, frequency, and healing. These invisible yet profoundly powerful agents are consequently more effective than the standard methods we commonly use for the same purpose. In the future, there is no doubt that we will alter cells and genes by guiding the mind into uncharted realms via advanced technologies. For five decades, I have employed state-of-the-art electromagnetic therapies in the conquest of helping people heal.

My biggest concern is the lack of interest and funding for these genius methods that rightfully need to be supported to advance the future of healthcare. Time can be both our friend and our foe, although it tends to force practical and effective procedures to the top of the pile. By more of us rallying behind future science, together, we can help to facilitate the birth of a new set of healing tools so that we may increase the opportunities for maintaining health beyond the limits of our current "health care systems."

CHAPTER 2:

History of Energy as a Tool

Reality is merely an illusion, albeit a very persistent one.
- Albert Einstein

"Although I am a typical loner in daily life, my consciousness of belonging to the invisible community of those who strive for truth, beauty, and justice has preserved me from feeling isolated."
- Albert Einstein

Carl Jung spoke about the evolutionary brain of humans in four categories. Primitive humans used the right side of their brains for maximum awareness. Ancient man slowly shifted toward their left hemisphere, and Modern man lost much of what primitive people inherently possessed (instinctual awareness). Today contemporary people are regaining the right hemisphere like our primal ancestors. Ironically, we always think of the original people as uncivil, savage, and unconscious. We now understand that they possessed a wide, comprehensive grasp of the interconnectedness of all life. They seemed to be at one with nature and the universe. As they broke out of their shells and began community via communication, it was the rhythm of drums that became language. Mimicking sounds and natural elements like fire, water, earth, and air, they proceeded to manifest a unified culture. Humbly embracing themselves as part of a larger tapestry, permitting them to rely on naturally occurring processes.

Slowly moving into the ancient human status, they became less intuitive and more cerebral. This formidably impacted their perception, developing unhealthy ego in the process. The mono-focused modern man has fooled himself into believing that he is the epicenter of all reality and independently capable of ruling the universe. This detachment from the ecological and cosmic systems that govern life makes him a nemesis to natural order. There now is an emerging group of contemporary humans that are recapturing the significant consciousness that our earliest human ancestors once possessed. For this reason, I think it fit to describe some of the bio-frequency powers used in the development of their societies.

Original humankind was sensitive to the bio-frequency fields of the earth (7.83 Hz) and the atmospheric changes that occurred throughout the seasons. Dowsing was consistently employed as a tool to reveal the geometric fields of energy hidden below the surface of the earth.[30] Homes, villages, towns, and cities were most often settled in areas that were either neutral or high-frequency vortexes. Places of worship, temples, churches, and synagogues were routinely built where the highest level of positive organized bio-geometry existed. Today, this is seldom discussed and even scoffed at by the intellectuals who have hijacked modern science. We, as researchers, should recognize that our obligation is to heighten our capacity to understand by fully observing what nature is doing with or without our knowledge.

Four decades ago, I brought an engineer to the acreage that Hippocrates has settled on. Fortunately, there was only a single vein of underground disruptive abnormal currents that, in this particular location, invisibly bisected a busy office where many of our team worked. One of our most committed and efficient employees sat in the area that was highly affected by this naturally occurring current. She said, "I found it difficult to sit still at my desk" until we grounded this disharmonious wave by installing copper wires that were geometrically shaped into neutralizing patterns and then positioned into the ground. None of the team was aware of this alteration, yet there was an immediate change in the way people felt and worked. Can you imagine how much disruption occurs globally since we do not acknowledge such powerful forces? We all stand at a pinnacle time in human history that can vault us into the higher realms of consciousness. Upon arriving, we will become acutely familiar with the energetic resources that abound on and around this beautiful planet on which we reside. We already possess the knowledge and abilities, and there are guides in the advanced sciences who can lead the way.

Our ancestors, as diverse as they were, created magnificence out of the wisdom of the cosmos. When primal man and two of his factions, Neanderthals and Homosapiens, were fighting for survival in Europe, one unique example of Sapiens, the Egyptians, were using sacred geometry to create their society and architectural marvels that we cannot replicate today. Indigenous tribes all over the planet have left behind structures, art, and rituals that allow us to comprehend the depth of awareness that they possess. Our guilt-ridden minds, with their awkwardness and arrogance, lead us to consider historic man as a lesser creature. There is no doubt in my mind that many of our forebears were far more advanced than we could ever imagine.

Explorers in the Invisible

In the 19th century, Viktor Schauberger, a naturalist, wrote about his observations of water.[31] Be it a river, stream, brook, waterfall, lake, or ocean. Vortexes seemed to organize the structure of the hydrogen and oxygen (H20). In the 21st century, our top astronomers and quantum physicists explain how the multiple universes and the way planets operate within the cosmic systems are based upon this vortex model. All life and movement seem to be either growing outward (expanding), or when degradation or demise occurs, it is a reversal (contracting). It is now clear that light manifests matter, but for this to occur, there has to be resistant electron force like an antiparticle. It may be a positron. We all conceptually know that pressure can create diamonds.

Leonardo Da Vinci in the late 15th and early 16th centuries, in a similar way, described the unification of energy and matter, which also guided his artistic expression. Nostradamus was, first and foremost, a physician who was instrumental in having clinicians clean and sterilize their hands and instruments before practicing medicine. He was better known for his ESP (Extrasensory Perception)[32]. His immense vision permitted him to view the invisible microbes that would actually cause infections. Many of his writings detailed what he equated as a mathematical pathway to the future. Following its essential rhythm, he formulated a process that allowed him to predict future events. Thomas Edison often spoke of how he tapped into knowledge during his sleep. His ability to go into REM patterns of deep relaxation abolished his mental limitation, which expanded his ability to reach beyond his own boundaries.

The Neocortex, the third and latest layer of the evolutionary triune brain, which presented itself about two million years ago, gives us a tool for foresight, hindsight, and, most importantly, insight. Seldom do we access this gift, and rarely does anyone spend much time there. With emerging new sound, light, and laser technologies, we will hopefully all become more familiar with this human asset so that we can expansively grasp and employ higher sources of knowledge. Spiritual teachers over millennia tapped into this reservoir of wisdom, allowing them to guide and encourage their apprentice to resist the reptilian (primitive brain) patterns or practices that modern civilization now wallows in.

Historically, there have been exceptional people who, when consciously arriving at the expanse of the universe, disseminated their discoveries to all of humankind. An example of one of the most advanced scientists was Nikola Tesla, born on July 10, 1856. This highly intelligent Serbian man moved to the United States in 1887 and designed alternating dash current (AC) electrical systems. This, as you know, rapidly became the preeminent power system. His genius was hijacked by some of the world's top tycoons, and he was relegated to strike out on his own. One of his greatest feats was his (AC) Hydroelectric power plant designed for

Niagara Falls. All during this productive time, while he manifested life-changing technologies, his heart and soul thought well beyond the wires and the energy that they facilitated. In the late 1800's he created the Tesla Coil, laying the foundation for wireless technology. His objective was to find the web of naturally occurring frequencies that covered and moved within the earth. The most shocking yet motivating event that propelled him toward his ultimate goal was Marconi's theft of Tesla's transmission tower technology. As a result of this unfortunate circumstance, he buffered himself by moving to Colorado, far from the Long Island, New York, laboratories he labored in. He was finally free of the unwanted influence of the money machine and limited thinking of the scientific community, able to expand and expound on his passionate pursuit. He eventually discovered the bio-geometric energy currents in the earth to tap into for free energy. This was certainly not embraced by what had now become the electric industry and its governmental protectors. Tesla spent his later years pondering future science but found very few who understood the enormous contribution he was offering. As a legacy, some advanced thinkers have created the Tesla Science Center. This prestigious group seeks to purchase his original laboratory, converting it into a museum that will display his brilliance. Their highest goal is to encourage the hearts and minds of the next generation of scientists who may well liberate us from our self-imposed cycles of deception.

On the cutting edge of this new frontier, is neuroscience mapping of the brain. We have now unlocked how matter becomes our minds. Giving us a picture of how mental activity arises from carefully orchestrated interactions among different parts of the brain. Recognizing that networks of electrical frequency create thought provokes the question as to why it has taken tens of thousands of years to develop. What we have found, in areas identified as hubs, is that they are in the exact locations that have expanded the most during this evolutionary process. These epicenters are up to 30 times the size as in macaques (other areas of the brain). For example, if you think of the structure of the brain (matter) as an orchestra, evolution increased the number of musicians in a section of the ensemble, fostering more intricate melodies. One masterful conductor is a young man we will now discuss.

Britain's Daniel Tammet[33] for the lack of a better term is described as a savant. His mental abilities and understanding of universal patterns is well beyond that of anyone in history. Physicians are grasping in the dark to label him with a condition, since it is unfathomable to consider that he may well be the most functional human that science has ever documented. Imposing on him the label of autism is nonsensical since autistic people have difficulties functioning socially. Daniel does not display any challenges in this area, and in fact, he is an author, a speaker, and sought-after in the areas of mathematics, physics, and the biological sciences. His brain chemistry is able to manifest mathematical equations that supersede the most advanced computers. As if this were not enough, his language skills are earth shattering. Within seven days, he is able to study, learn, and articulate fluently even the most difficult languages. To reduce his so-called gifts to the function of the organ we call the brain would be a grand injustice. My understanding of Mr. Tammet's ability is that he has abolished the walls of limitation. On a conscious level, he taps into the omnipresent library that contains all knowledge. Many call members of his generation that possess exceptional intellect, Indigo Children. On a practical level we may note that the youngest members of our family are generally the most capable and competent with electronics. My two year old grandchild is significantly more sophisticated than I am in this area.

Are we on the brink of embracing a new way of thinking that will unshackle our inner genius from the imposition of limited conceptualization? Will we be able to communicate and create by sourcing our imagination and realizing it in a real world function? Today's technological geniuses tell us that the gap between concept and creation will become much smaller as we surge forward into the future. We believe that future quantum humans will be able to conceptualize and realize instantaneously. Previously this would have been considered magic, yet considering that all matter is energy, if we can drop the physical facade and move energy without the confines of structure, instantaneous manifestation is possible.

In our work at the Hippocrates Health Institute, shifting of one's negative mindset is the core tool we utilize in helping people eradicate disorders by visualizing their desired state of health. Time and time again, we have observed spontaneous remissions when imagination becomes reality. What an exciting time it is for the liberated professional scientists who are abandoning the norms of their training. This new frontier as all previous frontiers, is accepting, inviting, and brimming with endless possibilities. In the recent past, it was unthinkable for us to consider a machine that possessed virtual reality. Now let us as humans create a seamless, successful, actual reality.

Top scientists today are creating computer generated networks and subjecting them to evolutionary pressures, which ultimately could manifest advanced artificial intelligence (AI). What this means to the future of mankind is that we could actually resolve problems that the mind does not know exists. The next phase will be applying this to brain training, ultimately resolving the negative pathways and impulses that create all disorder and even physical disease. We are no longer jailed by the lack of knowledge about consciousness. This phenomenon is currently being charted so that it can be successfully employed by our descendants.

An important area of scientific endeavor is research which is leading us to better understand vision. The nodes of the Inferotemporal (IT) cortex are in both brain hemispheres. This is a cerebral realm which identifies faces. As science is dissecting the electrical impulses that move from the iris to these middle Lateral and middle Fundus areas, we are patching together the extraordinarily elaborate processes allowing us to recognize familiar people, places, and things. Our electrically charged neurons (brain and nerve cells) are fully capable carriers of data and information.

Of course, with all of this advanced probing into the functionality of our brain awareness and our interaction with all else, man has begun to tinker in a dangerous way. Implanting brain devices, which has already been done by the US military, funded with more than seventy million tax dollars, throws a figurative wrench into the positive benefits derived by utilizing the electrical system instead of the biochemical body. These bio-meds are called electroceuticals and/or bio-electronics. Among this new area of "Frankenscience" are digital pills, called Abilify MYCite[34], (anti-psychotics), which contain sensors that are the size of a grain of sand. These nano devices are activated when they come in contact with stomach acid. The sensors send a signal to a patch that has been affixed atop the rib cage, which then sends data to an "App." This is a technological way, abused to continually dose patients, allowing physicians / psychiatrists to profit by up to eight thousand dollars more, per patient per year. On the other end of the spectrum, when this diagnostic tool is humanly employed, it may help to prevent a wide spectrum of disease. Data, such as time of consumption and release of medicines or body chemistries (such as body pH, microbial activity, and cancer cell development, etc...), can all be monitored.

Light and Sound

Ancient cultures worshipped the sun and thought of it as the umbilical cord to life. From this grew multitudes of color and light therapies spanning from the Ayurvedic treatments in color light boxes to the subliminal therapeutic lighting that John Ott contributed in Disney's film, Fantasia. Dr. Jacob Lieberman explains in his contribution Light: Medicine of the Future,[35] that the rainbow colors that present themselves in the outdoor environment have therapeutic effects when they filter through our eyes and activate our body's and brain's harmonization processes. The mere act of exclusively wearing sunglasses and never taking in natural sun rays makes us more vulnerable to aging and disease. This sounds almost counter-intuitive since modern hypotheses on the subject place the sun in "bad light," almost as an enemy. As we expand forward, enlightening ourselves to the magnificent and genius of the biological, psychological and cosmic systems, we are recognizing and embracing all to be a gathering of frequencies, vibration, light, and sound. All of this creates what we know as reality.

Sounds are vibrations that are infinite and can be formed into thought, imagination, and music, the latter being an artistic expression of one's imagination. From the Mozart Effect, which enhances special reasoning in humans[36] and encourages infant brain development to promote plant growth via the application of classical music, we recognize the nourishing effect of suitable melodic stimulus. Our work at Hippocrates has wired the growing sprouts so that they together compose and perform musical concerts. In the twentieth century, Monroe revealed that certain notes created with electronics, cracked open deep memories and feelings to such a point, it became therapy. We all potentially harbor unresolved issues and traumas in our cells and organs. When we can break through the layers that conceal them, they are then released. This liberates emotional blockages that may be the culprit that holds you back.

There are few people on earth that have not experienced beautiful memories upon hearing music that is familiar. Love is expressed through assembling notes that universally touch others hearts with the composer's sentiment. As an example, these compilations of sounds may be used in parades to have participants all move in a rhythmic way. What would a movie be without the music, which actually plays the largest role in activating emotions?

We recently conducted a research study in coordination with the University of Florida on the viability of Wholetones Healing Frequency[37]. These electronic devices are used as sleep aides and calming therapies. Our objective is to find whether they have an impact on those people with insomnia. This sleep disorder has risen to a formidable concern for billions worldwide. Abnormal brain frequencies that are often provoked by stress, negative attitudes, hormones, and fear is a prominent instigator in the development of many disorders including premature aging.

CHAPTER 3:

Anatomy Of A 'Miracle'

The rare but spectacular phenomenon of spontaneous remission of cancer persists in the annals of medicine, totally inexplicable but real, a hypothetical straw to clutch in the search for cure.
- Caryle Hirshberg[38]

It only takes an instant for someone's life to be tragically altered by the vagaries of 'chance.' Twenty-one-year-old Mitchell May's life-changing moment came on a rain-slick highway in Tennessee as he and five friends were driving their Volkswagen van to a bluegrass music festival. Mitchell had swiveled around in the front passenger seat to hand his friends in the back some sandwiches he had made when suddenly an oncoming blue car began to spin out of control, skidding directly towards them.

The careening auto hit with tremendous force on the passenger side, collapsing the van and crushing it inward at the spot where Mitchell was sitting. He was catapulted feet-first through the windshield, his body hanging halfway out onto the hood. He lay there unconscious while rescuers spent 45 minutes frantically cutting through the metal that had twisted around him like a steel cocoon.[39]

No one else was seriously hurt, but Mitchell's injuries were life-threatening. By the time he was placed in an ambulance, his punctured lungs had collapsed, and his heart had stopped beating. The valiant ambulance crew restarted his heart and kept him alive while rushing him to the nearest hospital. For the next week, Mitchell remained in a coma as doctors assessed the seriousness of his multiple injuries. Aside from suffering numerous broken ribs, his left leg was broken in six places, and his right leg was so badly mangled that the doctors were certain it would require amputation.

When Mitchell finally regained consciousness, he found himself immersed in searing pain. The exposed nerves in his shattered right leg burned and ached constantly, undiminished by the shots of morphine and other painkillers. He was transported from the hospital to an intensive care ward at the state's largest medical facility in Nashville, where attending physicians concluded that he would never walk again without assistance even if they could save both legs, which was doubtful. They urged him to consent to an operation to remove his widely infected right leg. Though Mitchell still periodically lapsed into unconsciousness, he understood the gravity of his injuries and the grim long-term prognosis, yet he adamantly refused to allow any amputation. His physicians thought he was just being delirious, but Mitchell instinctively felt, without a sliver of doubt, that an option would be found to save his leg if he could hold out a while longer.

More than 2,000 miles away in Los Angeles, Mitchell's father, Marvin May, a professor at UCLA, arranged for his son to be admitted to the school's renowned Medical Center, where a prestigious team of vascular and orthopedic surgeons and other specialists had been assembled to treat him. Wearing a full body cast, a metal plate attached to pieces of his leg bone, and doped out of his mind, Mitchell was flown home to face the next challenging phase of his extraordinary ordeal.

Chief orthopedic surgeon Dr. Edgar Dawson had treated many severe injuries during his long career at UCLA as a Clinical Professor of Surgery.[40] Nothing compared to the gravity of the situation he faced with Mitchell May. Dr. Dawson's report on Mitchell's condition came right to the point: "Joints at the ankle and knee of the right leg have been destroyed. More than two inches of bone and nerve tissue in that leg have been torn away. From just below the knee down to the ankle, there is bare bone hanging out with no muscle or skin over it. There is a lot of tissue loss. There is oozing green fluid coming out of holes in the bone. The leg is grossly infected. It has to come off!"

Several dozen physicians and specialists examined Mitchell and concurred with Dr. Dawson's opinion – the leg must be removed, or the patient would die from the raging infection and blood poisoning. Despite this medical verdict and even a tearful plea from his family, Mitchell steadfastly refused the operation. Though the pain was so intense that it felt like "many dentists were simultaneously drilling into nerves sticking out of a hundred dental cavities," his bravery would not permit him to give up. He was certain that he would not only survive but would someday walk again on both legs.

Desperate to save their son's life, Marvin and Lorraine May were ready to take the medical staff's advice and sign a court order that would force Mitchell to undergo the operation. Lorraine decided at the last moment to attempt to fulfill her son's wishes. If there was any miracle to be summoned, maybe she had to place faith in her son's stubborn will to survive. She had heard about an unconventional research project underway in the University of California's psychology department. An experiment involving 'hands-on' healers was being conducted by Thelma Moss, PhD., a visionary psychology professor with an unusual resume.[41]

Professor Moss had entered academia following a successful career both as a movie screenwriter –her biggest hit being *Father Brown*[42], starring Alec Guinness in 1954-- and later as an author whose 1962 autobiographical book, *My Self And I*[43], became a bestseller by chronicling the treatment and psychological problems she experienced following her husband's death from cancer two days after she gave birth to her daughter. She had always been interested in the untapped powers of the human mind and when she joined the school's faculty, she carved out a special niche for herself by heading up UCLA's fledgling parapsychology[44] laboratory,[45] where she initiated investigations of human 'energy fields.'

When Lorraine May approached Professor Moss for help in saving the life of her son, Moss promptly recommended the services of a gifted healing practitioner who worked with her in the laboratory as a research assistant. His name was Jack Gray, a balding 65-year-old immigrant with a distinctive New York accent, a fondness for polyester leisure suits, a resemblance to the actor Fred Astaire, and a background just as colorful as Thelma Moss. Born in Austria, he was the seventh son of a seventh son, which in his family's Jewish Kabbalistic tradition meant he was a special child. After immigrating to New York, Jack played the clarinet in Vaudeville productions and got to know some of the yogis who laid on beds of nails and performed other mind-over-matter methods. From these mentalists, he learned how to enter trances to control his own physiology and other feats, which later would prove to be useful skills when he began his practice in Los Angeles.

Within a few hours of accepting Professor Moss's request to treat Mitchell as a research project, Jack said goodnight to his wife and children at his San Fernando Valley home, got behind the wheel of his wheezing Ford Pinto, and drove directly to the hospital. In an intensive care room, he found Mitchell, all five foot seven inches of him, still encased in the body cast and delirious with pain and a 104-degree fever. In the throes of his agony, Mitchell had jerked half the hairs out of his beard, which, to Jack, was a sure sign that he had to first work on relieving this unbearable torment.

Jack reached down and gently touched Mitchell's forehead and softly said, "Mitchell, you were made in the image and likeness of God. Everything you will ever need is within you."

Throughout the night until sunrise, without a break for sleep, without even sitting down, Jack's hands danced and moved rhythmically through the air three inches above Mitchell's injuries. He alternately recited prayers and used his voice to induce deep trance states in the young man.

At times, Jack released startling guttural sounds and hypnotic chanting, urging Mitchell to summon his own voice and marshal his energy to join in. For three consecutive nights, he tirelessly performed this ritual, often repeating to his patient: "You are created in the image and likeness of God; therefore, everything you need for healing is already within you! You can heal this leg! You will heal this leg!"

Even when Mitchell fell asleep from the medications, Jack continued with the work of reprogramming his subconscious. "You desire to be normal and natural, healthy and strong," Jack intoned. "You desire very much to save that leg by the power of your mind. By your own faith and belief and trust in yourself."

After the third session, Mitchell's unbearable pain, a pain that had defied the most powerful deadening agents that pharmaceutical medicine had to offer, began to subside until it completely disappeared. Baffled by what they were seeing, Mitchell's parents asked Jack, "What are you doing to our son?" The healing practitioner patiently explained how he was only playing the role of a facilitator, helping to restore Mitchell's life force, known in China as Qi[46] and in India as Prana[47], while reprogramming their son's subconscious so he could take on the task of healing himself by harnessing the regenerative powers of his own immune system.

Dr. Dawson was impressed with what he was witnessing. As he confessed to Mitchell's parents, "Your son had pain in his right leg from causalgia, which is one of the most painful conditions known. It's a nerve pain and science has not determined its source, offering no effective treatment[48]. I don't know if it was the 'mind-power healing,' the suggestions, or what, but something stopped Mitchell's causalgia, and it abruptly stopped. I have absolutely no idea how his pain went away on its own."

As the months went by and Jack continued the healing sessions, Mitchell's infection disappeared, and his life was no longer in jeopardy. Most remarkable of all, he began to regenerate skin, muscle, nerves, and bone in the wounded leg. The two-inch gap started filling in with new bone. Additionally, missing muscle tissue and nerves appeared, and the fractures that were beyond repair began to fuse. This alignment and knitting together of leg bones was occurring despite having never been set by physicians. The healing effects were so unusual that Mitchell became like a living science experiment for doctors, researchers, and students at the Medical Center, who converged with regularity to whisper among themselves while marveling at his steady, regenerative progress.

Mitchell graduated from a wheelchair to walking with crutches and a brace, then discarded these and began strolling on his own without assistance. The physicians who had treated him shook their heads and rolled their eyes with disbelief. Upon examining x-rays of Mitchell's nearly healed right leg, Dr. Dawson was awestruck and blurted out: "I never would have believed it possible, but he has reformed an ankle bone!" Not only that, but his tibia regenerated nearly two inches of bone, which had been thought to be medically impossible.

In his conversations with other physicians, Dr. Dawson would often describe Mitchell's recovery as nothing short of mind-boggling. "I can tell you that it was not me that got Mitchell to where he is functioning today. Mitchell's leg was gone. There was no hope of saving it. I had scheduled him for amputation. People who have this serious wound never get better. It just doesn't happen. But it did in his case. What else can we call it but a miracle?"

By 1976, just four years after his devastating accident, Mitchell had not only regained full use of his right leg, enabling him to walk normally and to go dancing with his girlfriend, but he also undertook more rigorous activities, including a four-week-long hiking trip into the wilderness, and a climb into and out of the Grand Canyon carrying a heavy backpack along the steep trails. People who didn't know his remarkable history would not have suspected that this vital young man had once been facing imminent death and, at best, classified by conventional medicine as someone hopelessly crippled for life.[49]

Other than Dr. Dawson, none of the medical professionals involved in Mitchell's case ever questioned Jack Gray about his healing techniques. None showed any interest in how he helped to end Mitchell's pain and assisted in regenerating his body. These were matters they preferred to file away as anomalies, something so far beyond the norm, a case so reeking of 'hocus pocus' and so resistant to replication in anyone else that it should be closed and forgotten forever. What they really felt and were reacting to was the peculiar professional anxiety that erupts from confronting the limits of their own knowledge and training.

Shortly before his injury occurred, Mitchell had been reading about the role that nutrition plays in maintaining health and rejuvenating the immune system. That interest was rekindled during his recovery, and Jack assisted him in gathering herbs, mushrooms, algae, and other natural and organically-grown plants to create specially blended 'superior living-food formulas' that worked synergistically to support his healing process. He used a bioenergy research camera in Dr. Moss' laboratory to capture the electromagnetic imprint, or life-force energy, of these various plants, selecting those for his own use that generated the most intense film signatures. All of them turned out to be botanicals commonly employed by traditional physicians of tribal societies who recognized their restorative properties.

Prior to Jack's death, he had been mentoring Mitchell and teaching him energy techniques to help other people. Mitchell also went back to college, got his Master's degree, opened a practice as a licensed psychotherapist, and initiated research into ways to measure healing energies as part of a postgraduate program at UCLA. Mastering a technique that combined the laying on of hands, nutrition, meditation, breathing exercises, and counseling, Mitchell's reputation spread until he no longer had the time to devote to private clients, so he held seminars to teach others how to heal themselves.

Mitchell explained, "We heal ourselves all the time, yet this takes place at an unconscious level. I teach my clients to breathe in a manner that activates healing energy. And we use methods to create space to go outside the inner islands that most of us inhabit. When we learn to enter into a conscious and participatory relationship with this inherent healing space, we tap into extraordinary possibilities. My own recovery is a testament to that."

Trying to separate and measure the efficacy of hands-on healing, the powers of suggestion and belief, the setting of intention, the placebo effect, and nutrition would be an impossible task. Obviously, his recovery process was not a double-blind randomized controlled lab study of the sort demanded by medical science as proof for any "so-called" medical claim; the lessons taken from his experience must necessarily be subjective and anecdotal. His recovery fits a pattern in which radical regeneration often appears to be a synergistic effect produced by many factors interacting together to amplify the inherent healing force of nature residing in every human being.[50] This force, no doubt, is a gathering of emotionally provoked and biologically existing subtle frequency, woven together with others, connecting all living things, unbounded by time.

Since the early seventies, I have been observing an unbroken chain of comprehensive healing and recoveries from cases modern medicine called "incurables." Seemingly these victims of disease tapped into an inner reserve that provided the power in increments that abolished the disorder that was threatening their lives. Unquestionably, all of us possess the absolute ability to reestablish health and wellbeing via Quantum Human Biology.

How Often Does Radical Regeneration Occur?

Probably the first rigorous and wide-ranging attempt to determine the frequency of spontaneous healings and 'miraculous remissions' came in 1993, with the publication of a study titled "Spontaneous Remission: The Spectrum of Self-Repair."[51] It was conducted by two scientific researchers at the Institute of Noetic Sciences, the California science research think tank founded by a former Apollo astronaut and moonwalker, Dr. Edgar Mitchell[52].

With more than 3,500 references from more than 800 medical and science journals in 20 different languages, the compendium constituted the largest database of medically reported cases of remission ever compiled anywhere in the world. Around 74 percent of the cases involved cancer; however, in the study, authors emphasized that both cancer and non-cancer remissions, along with miraculous recoveries from injuries, were vastly under-reported in medical literature because such cases are "often regarded as a conundrum created by the misdiagnosis of the patient's condition." Many physicians fear criticism from their peers in reporting unconventional remission cases, much less any seemingly miraculous medical phenomena ascribed to faith or an alternative remedy.

This study contrasted 'miraculous' remission with 'spontaneous' consistency and described unexpected and remarkable healings as being "sudden, complete and without medical treatment." The study reported, "These cases appear to involve some of the same pathways as (spontaneous) remission. However, consideration should be given to the possibility that the altered states of prayer, religious faith, and meditation may allow the process of self-repair greater freedom to operate. By contrast, so-called spontaneous remissions usually happen gradually over time, rather than suddenly, and are defined here as "the disappearance, complete or incomplete, of a multitude of diseases, including cancer, without medical treatment or treatment that is considered inadequate to produce the resulting disappearance of disease, symptoms, or tumors."[53]

The study authors discovered that even in conservative medical journal articles, physicians occasionally concede their lack of understanding in unique spontaneous remissions, proposing explanations that may credit 'alternative' treatments embraced by the patient. Here is a partial list:

--Under the term of 'psycho-spiritual,' which presumably included prayer and the 'laying-on-of-hands,' physicians found there to be remissions for pancreatic, nasopharynx, testis, breast, and bone sarcoma cancers.

--Meditation which was identified in medical journals as possibly being responsible for remissions in lung and bronchial cancers, bone sarcomas, breast, and colon cancer.

--Radical changes in diet, usually involving herbs and uncooked plant-based foods, constituted another category of alternative treatments linked to remissions of malignant melanomas, uterus cancer, bone sarcoma, breast and liver cancers.

The database of cases is divided into 19 categories of remission, such as neoplasms (abnormal proliferation of cancer cells) of the digestive organs, female breast diseases, nervous system and endocrine glands, infectious and parasitic diseases, respiratory and circulatory system maladies, and injury-related disorders. These cases are fascinating to read, even though the dry clinical descriptions do not express how remarkable the recoveries had truly been. Under infectious diseases, 12 cases of AIDs are described, in which the patients spontaneously reverted from positive to negative blood readings without any trace of the HIV remaining. One of the cases involved a two-year-old boy whose HIV infection, inherited from his mother, was accompanied by persistent pneumonia and suddenly disappeared for no apparent reason.[54]

Perhaps the most extraordinary category was summarized in a 1983 medical journal article documenting 13 cases of spontaneous recovery by people in the U.S. who had been declared legally blind. Their blindness had resulted from a disease called Presumed Ocular Histoplasmosis Syndrome, which is known as an 'incurable' malady that produces lesions robbing people of their eyesight. By staid medical standards, an article in The *International Ophthalmology Clinics* journal used awestruck language, reporting "the exceptional return of vision" in these patients and the mystery of this "spontaneous recovery phenomenon."[55]

Many so-called spontaneous remissions are not really spontaneous – except perhaps from the physician's point of view—because the patients were working hard for the remission to occur by using unconventional healing methods like self-administered Reiki, self-hypnosis, or visualization. There also seem to be certain types of remissions that are purely biological, caused by infections and fevers that provoke the immune system into taking sudden and dramatic action. Some cancers emerge by evading the recognition radar of the immune system until the cancer growth is out of control. A raging fever in the body, either by coincidence or if intentionally induced (hyperthermia), might wake up the immune system and in the process of fighting this fire, the system discovers and combats the cancer.

A more limited attempt at measuring the incidence of remission in cancer came in a study published by the American Cancer Society journal, *Cancer*, which examined cases of non-small cell lung cancer, an 'incurable disorder' with an average survival rate after diagnosis of just six months. The researchers found that about one percent of those diagnosed went on to live for five years or more (some were completely healed) without any medical treatment other than tiny doses of radiotherapy to relieve symptoms, such as growths, from the malignancy.[56]

One theory offered is that these surviving patients are "astonishingly sensitive to low doses of radiation," in the words of Professor Michael MacManus[57], an Australian radiation oncologist who co-authored the study. The study states: "There is evidence that low-dose radiation to cells can actually have a greater effect than bigger doses. There's also evidence that very low doses of radiation can actually improve the survival of a cell."[58]

In this study, we are introduced to what will be a recurrent theme in this book --- tiny doses of something (in the case of a placebo, a dose of 'nothing' or a suggestion) can set in motion huge biochemical changes in the human body. Greatly diluted portions of a chemical or healing agent leave a subtle 'shadow' in blood that provokes a healing response in the body. In the realm of chemical toxicity, science researchers acknowledge that endocrine-disrupting synthetic chemicals cause highly toxic effects, even at extraordinarily low doses in the one-part-per-billion range (equal to extensive sun exposure).[59] Take the placebo effect, for example, which might even, in part, explain homeopathy. It is a whole lot of nothing, yet it is a powerful force in healing, as I will document later in this book.

From this principle of 'less can be more,' the finding that low-dose radiation can possibly be advantageous reveals a possibility. It may be worth exploring whether reported 'energy' healings, remissions, and radical regeneration that are low-level transfers of a subtle form of energy (from practitioner to patient) can trigger the body's own inner healing powers. These practitioners don't 'harbor' this frequency; they tap into it from the omnipresent field that governs the multiverse. Energy exists in every element of our world and the universe.[60] We can be in tune with this ever-present energy to heal ourselves.

CHAPTER 4:

An Energy Affecting Humans and Animals

"The secret of change is to focus all of our energy not on fighting the old, but on building the new...the energy of mind is the essence of life." - Aristotle (384-322 BC)

Our bodies and those of animals are surrounded by an electromagnetic field. It is measurable as a pivotal method. In 2008, researchers at the Department of Anatomy at the Indiana University School of Medicine conducted this research titled "Distant Healing of Small-Sized Tumors."[61] Thirty mice were injected with cancer cells. Each day, a biology student in a white lab coat performed a 'treatment,' using only her hands and directed intention, and focused on a mouse inside its plastic cage. Only six days earlier, the cancerous tumor on the belly of one mouse had been so large that it could barely move, but the tumor had shrunk to half its former size, and the mouse had regained its vitality. All of this was apparently due to the treatment it was given. The treatment was an exchange of energy (love and care) that has electromagnetic fields that we share for self-healing.

The lab assistant had been trained to feel compassion for this tiny creature. She began the session by placing her hands on either side of the cage. For a few moments, she kept her mind blank, clearing it of judgment and negative thoughts. Her emotional intent of caring was transmitted to the mouse.

She and her fellow lab assistants had been picked by Margaret Moga[62], an associate professor in this Department. Professor Moga was an expert on rodents, with a Ph.D. from Loyola University's Chicago Medical Center. Her interest in alternative approaches to healing developed as a result of a positive personal experience she had with moxibustion, a 1000-year-old Asian medical therapy for arthritic joints[63]. This healing process involved burning an herb called moxa over the area of inflammation. That experience using an ancient remedy, one often disparaged by her medical colleagues as a worthless superstition, had given Professor Moga an open mind about experimenting with other healing traditions.

As the lab assistants held their palms over the mouse in each of their sessions, they rapidly cycled a series of images through their minds. These images were generated by personal lists the lab assistants had prepared prior to the experiment. They each had written down 20 outcomes they wanted in their lives, specific goals that involved other people, their own health, ideal jobs, mates, or material aspirations. Every item on the list was translated into images that represented the achievement of that goal. For example, if a person had an injured back but wanted to attain a certain back-bending yoga position, he or she visualized being effortlessly in that position, rather than visualizing a successful surgery to fix their back. Thus, each of the images was created as a symbol unique to that person.

These images were memorized, and the assistants practiced cycling them, like a continuous movie in their minds, no matter what conflicting feelings and emotions they might have. While the cycling of these images went on, the lab assistants imagined an energy flowing out of the palms of their hands and into the caged mice. For example, people who study yoga or tai chi use the energy flowing through their twelve meridians to accomplish posture and movements which confirms the flow of energy in humans and animals.[64] Fifteen mice were a part of the experimental group receiving direct 'treatments' after cancer cell exposure. Another 15 mice composed the control group and received no direct attention, after being injected with cancer cells. Also, a third group of 25 mice were age-matched controls and did not receive injections. All three of these groups lived in cages in separate rooms of the facility on the school's campus.

As the experiment unfolded, five animals from each group were examined at 5, 9, and 13-week intervals. Their blood hemoglobin levels were measured, and their spleens were weighed at each stage to determine whether their immune systems had been activated.

The age-matched group without cancer had marginally lower hemoglobin levels, but "significantly' lower spleen weights than the experimental and control groups. At 12 weeks, for instance, the experimental mice had spleens *three times* the weight of the age-matched group. The researchers italicized their published findings for emphasis; "*At weeks 9 and 13, there was no significant difference between the experimental and untainted control groups.*" None of the mice in either the experimental group or the two control groups had cancerous tumors, though only the experimental group had received the 'treatments.'

Based on everything traditional oncologists know or think they should know about cancer and mortality, all 30 of the cancer-injected mice in both the control and experimental groups should have died. The tumors that normally would grow quickly on their bodies after injection with cancer cells should have crushed their internal organs. After being injected with fatal doses of mouse mammary adenocarcinoma tumor cells, the resultant malignancies should have killed 100 percent of subjects within 14 to 27 days after injection.[65]

That is what had *always* happened during cancer drug experiments when cancer cells were introduced into mice. The same thing *should* have happened this time. No experimental drug of any sort was being used. The only 'treatment' being performed at all was the physical presence of lab assistants trained to project life-affirming visual imagery.

None of the 'treated' mice died of the cancer! Each one lived out its normal lifespan. Not only that, but both the control and experimental groups of 15 mice experienced similar survival rates, a phenomenon that the researchers speculated was due to bio-energy fields or resonance field theories. It seemed that a 'scatter effect' had occurred when the lab assistants projected their regenerative intentions. Historically, this is commonly known as the 100th Monkey Theory.

When some of the fully recovered study mice were later injected with more cancer cells, without any accompanying energy 'treatment,' they *did not* develop cancer. They had apparently evolved immunity to a disease that is a common scourge of humankind.

If these test subjects had been humans, who were the subjects of a cancer study, we might ascribe this as their miraculous, spontaneous remissions to the power of suggestion and the mysterious placebo effect. However, conscious or unconscious expectations of remission cannot be induced in mice, at least as far as we know, so there must have been an activation of their immune systems by an alteration in their energy fields. A hint of how this mechanism might work came in a second experiment, also by Moga, that detected low-frequency magnetic field oscillations in the vicinity of the treated mice cages. (This anomaly will be explored in a later chapter.) The study results, co-authored by Professor Moga and Professor William Bengston of St. Joseph's College in New York, were published in the April 2007 edition of the peer-reviewed *The Journal of Alternative and Complementary Medicine*.[66] This was called a replication experiment because it successfully duplicated the results of four previous studies that used the same cancer treatment protocols. These previous studies also produced data about 'bio-energy resonance fields,'[67] an evolving theory that all life is linked in an intricate web of influences operating at the quantum level. This, too, will be detailed in a later chapter.

The four studies conducted on mice and bio-energy healing since 2000 were conducted at New York's Queen's College and St. Joseph's College under Professor Bengston's research leadership. In the first study, published in the Journal of Scientific Exploration[68], Bengston himself became an apprentice to learn the 'laying on of hands' technique so he could participate in the study he had designed.

At the Brooklyn campus of St. Joseph's College, the skeptical chairwoman of the biology department, Professor Carol Hayes, selected three biology major volunteers to be trained as energy conductors for one of the studies. All three volunteers were non-believers in the legitimacy of this as a healing technique. In an added twist, each volunteer also took an experimental mouse home for daily treatments once the cancer cells were injected.

Four control mice were sent to a distant city. All died within the expected 27-day period. However, all of the mice taken home by the volunteers went into remission from the cancer, as did two mice in the laboratory group. The remission pattern seen in the mice was the same in all of these experiments. After a tumor had developed, an encrusted area on its surface emerged as healing progressed. Subsequently, the mouse's body began to reabsorb the tumor in a process that would result in the complete disappearance of the malignancy. That might help to explain why, in the later Moga experiment, it was found that the mouse spleens had tripled in weight, though the enlarged spleens were free of cancer.

The remission rates for each of the four studies defied all conventional assumptions about survival rates. In the first experiment, five of five experimental mice remitted; experiment two saw 7 of 7 in complete amelioration; experiment three had 7 of 10 remit; experiment four documented 10 of 11 in remission.

As the published study in 2000 further noted, "Perhaps most persuasively, we were unaware that the experimental biologist at St. Joseph's College had re-injected several remitted mice months after the experiments were over. *Without further treatment, these mice were immune to the mammary adenocarcinoma.*"

In one of Professor Bernard Grad's experiments at Canada's McGill University, he tested whether human hands and the subtle energy emanating from them could accelerate healing in mice.[69] He and his assistants took 48 wounded mice and placed them in three groups of 16 each: the first (the control group) was given no treatment; the second group received contact from a healer's hands, while the third group was only exposed to heat comparable to that of a healer's hands.

Over a period of 30 days, the wounds were monitored for recovery. Results showed that abrasions on the mice in the healer-treated group had either healed completely or were very tiny and nearly healed. Mice in the healer-treated group also evidenced a much faster rate of wound healing.

Grad's results were replicated using a larger group of 300 mice by G.I. Paul and Remi Cadoret, at the University of Manitoba. The big difference was these researchers used randomly selected individuals to apply the hand 'treatments,' as opposed to persons who claimed to have energy-healing abilities. These results with mice prompted me to raise a series of questions that ultimately became guideposts for this book.

If skeptical and inexperienced people can be taught to use a simple technique to achieve 90 percent and more remission rates in mice, what would be the impact of these healing influences on humans who have cancer and other diseases? How effective could such techniques be in maintaining our own immune systems for optimal preventative health? A place to start in the search for answers might be a review of the expansive human experience with this healing force of nature.

Hippocrates developed the comprehensive cancer program as a multi-team approach that focuses centrally on visualizing the desired reversal that a person conjures in their heart and mind. This mindfulness approach has been successfully employed for millennia, yet it is only recently that numerous scientific studies have validated the biological effect it creates in strengthening the immune system's cells that effectively search out and destroy all forms of cancer.

CHAPTER 5:

Reaffirming Ancient Healing Principles

"Every feeling is a field of energy; a pleasant feeling is an energy which can nourish. Irritation is a frequency which can destroy."
- Thich Nhat Hahn, Vietnamese Thi☐n Buddhist monk, celebrated teacher, peace activist, poet, and prolific author.

Ancient healing practices always included several natural methods and local herbs and spices. Self-healing, using the power of ritual and suggestion, and the healing of others by the 'laying-on-of-hands' can be traced back thousands of years in accounts of healers in ancient civilizations. Globally, tribal cultures also practiced indigenous healing methods[70]. We are familiar with the many historical accounts.

Perhaps the most famous claims of hands-on healing are found in the New Testament descriptions of Jesus and his healing ministry. He is said to have touched Peter's mother-in-law to cure a fever (Matthew 8:14-15); his hands healed a man with leprosy (Mark 1:40-42); by touch he healed two blind men (Matthew 20:29-34); with touch he restored hearing and speech in a man (Mark 7:32-35). Jesus also reputedly taught that, with faith and belief in him, these healing skills could be learned by anyone: "I tell you the truth, anyone who has faith in me, can do the same miracles I have done, and even greater things than these will you do." (John 14:12).

"It is believed by expert doctors that the heat which oozes out of the hand, being applied to the sick, is highly salutary. It has often appeared, while I have been soothing my patients, as if there was a singular property in my hands to pull and draw away from the affected parts aches and diverse impurities, by laying my hand upon the place, and extending my fingers toward it. Thus, it is known to some of the learned that health may be implanted in the sick by certain gestures and by contact." - Hippocrates (5th century B.C. Greek physician)

Practitioners of conventional Western medicine today view Hippocrates as the 'father' of medicine primarily because he took gods and demons out of the healing equation, replacing superstition with natural explanations for diseases and their 'cures.'[71] Alternative medical practitioners take a similar but more literal view of Hippocrates' legacy. They keep their focus on his belief that 'cures' for illness and disease come most readily from nature but require direct participation from the patient. There is no argument that healing comes from within.

It is debatable whether the 18th-century Austrian physician Franz Mesmer was more a charlatan than a genius. However, it is indisputable that he inspired developments in medicine that remain in common use more than three centuries later. The practice of hypnosis, for instance, and the employment of blue-ribbon scientific committees (today known as peer-reviewed) were used, and even the intentional use of placebos as a healing strategy. Mesmer hypothesized that magnets could cure illness. During his testing of the idea, he claimed to have discovered that a healer's own "animal magnetism" could be transferred into patients via magnets. The touching and stroking of the patient's body and the waving of his hands in a way that induced trances and cathartic release altered their state of mind, which we now know was activating an immune response.[72] 'Cures' of everything from fevers to paralysis were proclaimed everywhere he practiced. Pursuing ever greater glory and wealth, he moved to Paris. He created a sensation that attracted the attention of France's King Louis XVI, who appointed a commission of eminent scientists to investigate whether Mesmer and his healings were fraudulent.

Headed by the American ambassador to France, Benjamin Franklin (a pioneer in the study of electricity), and the other members of what may have been humanity's first blue-ribbon scientific commission, included Joseph de Guillotin (a physician whose invention of the guillotine would end the life of his employer) and Antoine Lavoisier, a famed chemist. They watched Mesmer in action, carrying out experiments on 'mesmerized' patients, and interviewed people who claimed Mesmer cured them of their ills. The commission's verdict was unanimous that animal magnetism did not exist. Still, the reported healings were genuine and resulted from the patient's imagination stoked by the power of suggestion induced by Mesmer. "Imagination without magnetism produces convulsions," read their report, "but magnetism without imagination produces nothing." Strangely, these giants in the field of 18th-century science and medicine failed to pursue the most intriguing and logical outgrowth of their findings – that medicine could harness suggestion and imagination to advance the cause of healing. They had inadvertently identified the placebo effect.

Mesmerism practices spread from Europe to the United States and inspired the idea that 'mind cures' could be developed to treat the afflictions of humankind. Maine clockmaker Phineas Quimby became adept at inducing trances in 1840 when he was 36 years old and attracted a following by reportedly healing people of paralysis, muteness, and other ailments.[73] He became one of the first to use a trance to anesthetize a patient before surgery performed by a doctor. Quimby believed that electricity passing from healer to patient was responsible, a healing that worked through the mind, using the setting of positive intentions and the identification and correction of negative beliefs in the patient. Any medicine can cure, insisted Quimby, "because the cure is not in the medicine, but in the confidence of the doctor." To one patient, Quimby declared; she must have faith in her own recovery because a cure "depends on your faith and your faith is what you receive from me."

During the American Civil War, Quimby was visited by a frail and sickly New Hampshire woman. She was 41-year-old Mary, who received his treatments. At the time, Quimby called his practice the "Science of Health," tapping into the healing "God within," which he said every human being possessed. Before he died in 1866, he was calling his healing approach "Christian Science."

Two weeks after his death, Mary fell on an icy street and suffered a concussion. During her recovery, while reading passages from the Bible describing the healing ministry of Jesus, she allegedly felt a divine revelation come over her, spontaneously healing her of her injuries.

Mary Baker Eddy attributed her 'recovery' to Quimby's Christian Science and set about writing a book on faith healing that she titled *Science and Health*[74]. When the book was published in 1875, it launched a new theological sect that culminated in the founding of the Church of Christ, Scientist. The key idea in her healing philosophy was that illness and disease are the consequences of wrong thinking and that 'cures' can be invoked by faith and a healthy attitude. By the early part of the 20th century, Christian Science had become the fastest growing denomination in the nation, reaching 200,000 practitioners, two-thirds of them women drawn mostly from the Methodist and Congregational churches. This emergence alarmed most physicians and even prompted humorist Mark Twain to write of his fear that the new religion was a dangerous cult intent on taking control of the U.S. Congress.[75]

"He would develop a sense of being positive within his own body, sickness being negative. He would draw his hands over the area of the pain and with a sweeping motion stand aside, shaking his hands and fingers vigorously, taking away the pain as if it were drops of water." - Grandson of D.D. Palmer (founder of Chiropractic Medicine)

Another 'magnetic healer' from this era whose practice is still widely disseminated today is D.D. Palmer[76], born in Toronto, Canada, whose grandson would one day describe his grandfather's healing technique this way:

After nine years of practicing this form of healing, Palmer decided that he would also begin manipulating the bodies of his patients to enhance their physiological well-being, and thus the new practice of chiropractic (meaning 'done by hand') was born. This technique in part was borrowed from already existing osteopathic methods.

The founder of modern psychology, William James, further contributed to this emerging field of mind-over-matter medicine. James called his practice the mind-cure religion of healthy-mindedness, which came from the International New Thought Alliance. This alliance was founded on the idea that Jesus Christ used the power of mind in his healing ministry. Ever since that time, methods employed by medical practitioners have been greatly reliant on placebos.

A farm boy from Maine named Ernest Holmes, who had been influenced by Baker Eddy's philosophy (self-healing & belief), wrote his own book, *The Science of the Mind*[77]. This book was published in 1926, which further elaborated on the idea that the unfettered mind can heal the body using affirmations and prayer. His book became the founding text in 1949 for The Church of Religious Science.[78] In more recent times, *Saturday Review* magazine editor Norman Cousins wrote a series of bestselling books, the first being *Anatomy Of An Illness* in 1979. This contribution chronicled his use of positive attitudes, faith, love, hope, and laughter inspired by Marx Brothers movies. 'Curing' himself of a debilitating and degenerative condition impelled him to share his discovery. These books were devoid of religious trappings or spiritual emphasis, yet still trumpeted the theme that the biochemistry of positive thought and human emotions, particularly when spiced with laughter, provide a key to any person's success in fighting illness and disease. Though Cousins was merely a journalist, not a physician or scientist, he was named an Adjunct Professor of Medical Humanities at the University of California School of Medicine[79]. There, he conducted research on the biochemistry of human emotions and healing until his demise.

Many alternative healing ideas and practices got their debut before a mainstream English-speaking audience in 1972 when *Time* magazine published an article titled "Faith, Hands and Auras,[80]" based on the proceedings of a conference at Stanford University that explored the emerging field of "parapsychological medicine." That conference drew 400 doctors, engineers, and biophysicists. The four-day event hosted 'faith healers' like Olga Worrall, acupuncture presentations, and biofeedback techniques. There was even Kirlian photography, which was employed by Thelma Moss at UCLA's Neuropsychiatric Institute to measure the electrical field (aura) surrounding all life forms. Auras are described as distinctive atmospheres or energy fields that surround and radiate from a person or object.

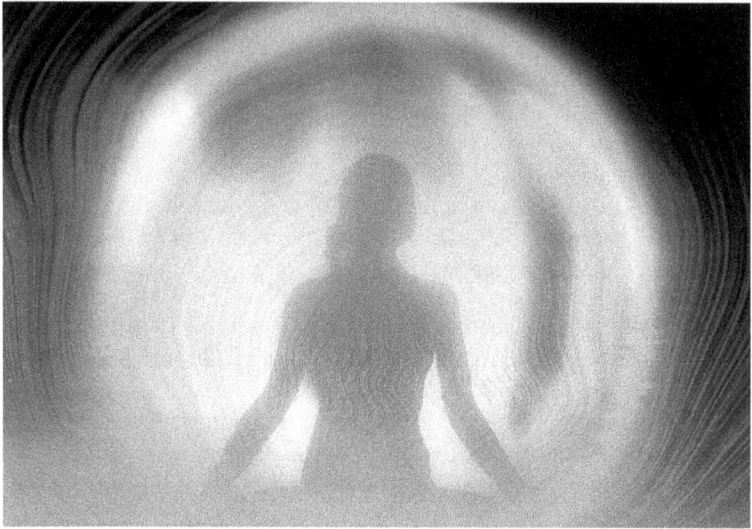

A few years ago, reports on the exploits of miracle workers would have drawn little more than scorn from scientifically trained individuals. However, many medical researchers are showing a newfound openness toward so-called psychic healing and other methods not taught in medical schools. Although it is vastly improved, it is premature to suggest that the majority of the scientific community is ready to accept **Quantum Human Biology**.

When confessed skeptics of unorthodox healing have, on occasion, evolved into ardent believers, it is usually because of their direct experience outside a classroom or laboratory, in which they observed radical regeneration firsthand. That path of transformation fits Gary E. Schwartz, Ph.D., a medical professor at the University of Arizona and director of its Laboratory for Advances in Consciousness. This Harvard-educated former Yale professor described in his 2007 book, *The Energy Healing Experiments*[81], three cases of 'energy healing' that he personally witnessed or had familiarity with, which opened his mind to the human potential that challenged his training and conventional worldview.

In the first case, Gary Schwartz watched a psychotherapist use her healing touch abilities to take away the pain of a man who had just broken his wrist. In the second, a New York woman had an ovarian tumor dissolved in a matter of weeks by a Reiki healer. Finally, and most remarkable of all, was a California man, hopelessly paralyzed from the neck down, who regained partial movement as a result of work done by a spiritual energy healer.

These healing miracles convinced Schwartz that "a collection of independently observed experiences begins to suggest that something real is going on and deserves scientific examination." To answer his own challenge, he initiated a series of human energy experiments over a decade, which I describe in a later chapter, using both trained healers and non-healers to pursue such questions as whether the human body projects invisible fields of energy and whether so, can people sense other people's energies? Can these energy fields be used to enhance healing and health?

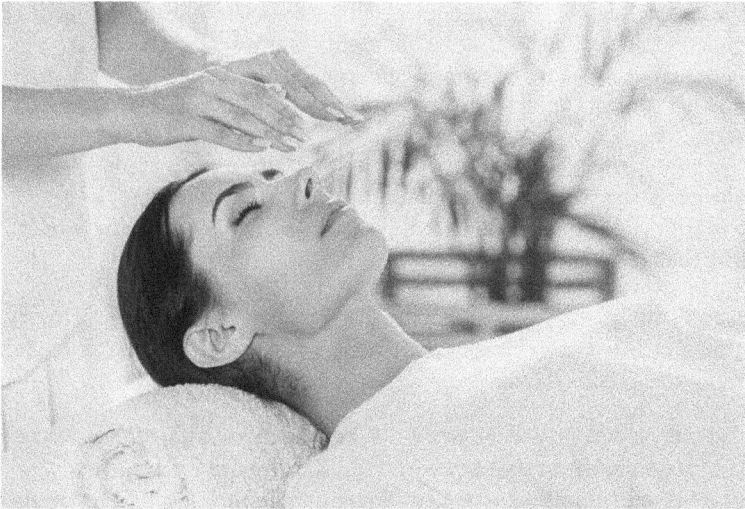

One battle line drawn in the scientific debate about unconventional healing has been over the very language used to label the phenomenon. What are we to call that healing force that works through an unknown, if not unknowable, mechanism? This force defies being pigeonholed into any prevailing theory about how consensus reality works. Among the culturally accepted (but scientifically disparaged) terms are energy healing, distance healing, energy medicine, prayer healing, vibrational healing, psychic healing, mind over matter, energy work, non-local mind, or healing intentionality.

Some practitioners and investigators of these phenomena do not concern themselves with precision in the language they use to describe the 'force' that apparently produces healing effects. Energy is a word often used promiscuously to mean a wide variety of things. That plays into the hands of critics, the scientific reductionist materialists, who note that only four kinds of energy are known to physicists –electromagnetic, gravitational, and the strong and weak nuclear forces—and, according to mainstream science, none of these have been conclusively shown to be responsible for healing effects recounted anecdotally, or allegedly observed in laboratory settings.

Without a theoretical model to explain such a phenomenon, committed skeptics are willing to discard the evidence for radical regeneration as anomalies produced by coincidence, wishful thinking, misperception, faulty experimental protocols, or, worse, fraud.

The absence of a working model for how these types of healing practices work should not necessarily be ammunition against the functionality of these practices. As the author of numerous books on healing and prayer, Larry Dossey, M.D., has pointed out,

"Although energy-based models may do quite well to explain what happens within the healer and healee, they don't work in explaining what happens in this invisible world between the healer and healee."[82]

In an essay he wrote for the journal, *Alternative Therapies*, Dr. Dossey (who prefers using the physics term 'non-local mind' for the phenomenon) elaborated on this theme:

"It is not lethal in science to admit ignorance about mechanism. This is particularly true in medicine, in which we often have known that something works before we understand the functional mechanism. For centuries we knew that drugs such as quinine, colchicine, and aspirin worked before we figured out how. We still don't know how general anesthetics work, but this fact has hardly limited their use."[83]

Some researchers have divided the dozens of alternative healing techniques and systems into a few broad categories:

- **Alternative Healing Systems** – Traditional Chinese medicine (including acupuncture); Ayurvedic medicine from India; and naturopathic and homeopathic medicine originating in Europe.
- **Manual Healing Techniques** – Chiropractic and Osteopathy (both developed in the U.S.), massage, reiki, qigong, etc.
- **Mind/Body Healing Techniques** – Biofeedback, hypnosis, meditation, prayer, visualization, etc.

Before leaving these fundamental areas, we cannot forget EMPATHS. There are many who say that 20% of the population is highly sensitive to others and their environment. Ambiance is a word that best suits their personality. It is often a double-edged sword to possess this hyper-receptivity since you can overthink, overreact, and overanalyze what is coming at you. Conversely, it affords you tools that can unlock consciousness that 80% or more of the population does not possess at a credible level.

This virtual radar is at some level in each person on Earth, although a defined percentage harbor enough to recognize it and employ it in their daily life. Many of the people mentioned above are most likely sophisticated empaths who refined their ability to utilize heightened perception in their exchange with others. Many of the so-called psychics are no more than seasoned empaths. ESP (extrasensory perception) is something that all of humanity possesses, yet few have refined their insightfulness to gain the pure messaging it offers.

Descriptions often used to describe these individuals are:

- **Clairsentient** - Hypersensitive emotions.
- **Clairaudient** - Clear Messaging.
- **Clairvoyant** - Multi Observational (vision).
- **Clairgustance** - Taste in fragrance sensitivity.
- **Claircognizance** - Sense of knowing.
- **Clairtangency** - Receiving information via touch.

Dr. Judith Orloff, MD, contributed a user-friendly guide called "The Empath's Survival Guide: Life Strategies for Sensitive People." [84] This literary work can help support those of you who feel a heightened sense of awareness that often overwhelms you. Be aware that much of what we call "mental illness" may not be just that but rather tsunamis of data that drown those who are not either prepared or aware of their gift.

For the purpose of this book, 'subtle bio-energies,' 'non-local quantum minds,' and other terminology are simply theories that underlie these alternative healing systems and techniques. I will use the term *Quantum Human Biology* to denote anomalous healing effects that have been documented in people and animals. It's really 'nature's innate healing force' that describes the mysterious energy mechanism producing those effects. Historically, Quantum technologies were used in scientific experiments in Physics.[85] Also, human biology is a widely studied subject matter in endless research. This book has combined these two major scientific methods to create *Quantum Human*.

CHAPTER 6:

Science Validates the Human Energy Field

Everything changes when you start to emit your own frequency rather than absorbing the frequencies around you; when you start imprinting your own intent on the universe rather than receiving an imprint from existence. - Barbara Marciniak

With all of the well-trained and academically conditioned minds over millennia, there has not been a consistent solid consensus on the construct of matter. The late Maurice Idels, who worked with numbers and endured the tough end of World War II, made an astonishing and highly plausible, as he calls it, "Nuclear Topology and The Blueprint of Matter." Also, the title of the 2024 book is one that I highly suggest serious seekers read.[86]

His remarkable insight is broken down in a simple way so that advanced science should engage in further research, solidifying this as a cornerstone contribution. Supersymmetry describes how nature effortlessly organizes all things into systems, patterns, and beautiful artistic imagery. Although this is measurable, it is made up of self-gauging constants. This is sub-particle science that goes deep beyond the atoms and neutrons into the world of geometric frequencies. He points out that energy densities from the electrons are manifested through subatomic particles that eventually become matter. These have been observed on rare occasions and labeled as Spinons and Holons.[87]

Although humanity has taken credit for the creation of mathematics, all that really happened is that we tapped into the already existing photonic energy that rains down from the sun. Multiverse-charged frequencies from the interactions of planets, the cosmos, and the constant eruption and change that lives within endlessly manifesting electrical connectivity that touches all things at all times in all cases. Occasionally, our ancestors would reference some of these higher conscious observations via words in the Hindu, Buddhist, Jewish, Muslim, Christian, and Baha'i theology. Many fine artists from cultures long gone drew these cosmic patterns into stunning imagery that still pleases us today.

For us to talk about our personal inner mechanics that connect us to all of this electrical charge and the perpetual universes, I think it is important to express that we, in great part, have the foundational understanding of how this scientifically works.

"Humans are electrical machines," wrote University of Oxford physiology professor Frances Ashcroft in her 2012 book, *The Spark of Life: Electricity in the Human Body*.[88] Light is inside us and the term "seeing the light" is a reflection of our truth and internal knowledge depicted as electricity. We unveil the evidence for this general truth every day. Consider when static electricity builds up in our bodies, such as when we walk on synthetic carpet, which jolts us as we touch a metal doorknob, or when a spark discharges with the touch of another person's hand. When a swimmer in the ocean is attacked by a shark, it is because the shark has detected the low-voltage electric field projected from the human's body. We are made of light and electricity, which manifests in our energy field that others may feel.

A chain of proteins called the ion channel accounts for the electrical activity of all nerves and muscles in your anatomy.[89] Each one of our sensory experiences are translated by these channels into electrical signals interpreted by the brain as sight, sound, and other sensations. The five senses (touch, feel, hear, see, and smell) are our primary sources of input received by the brain and translated into electrical signals which are transported via synapses.

We know that electricity is energy, yet, as Ashcroft pointed out in her research work, "there is a fundamental difference between the electricity that powers our bodies and that which lights our cities." Subatomic particles called electrons flow through the electrical wiring of our buildings. The currents in human and animal life are electrically charged atoms called ions. Four ions that are positively charged are sodium, potassium, calcium and hydrogen, and one negatively charged ion is chloride.

It is the movement (chemical transmission) of these ions across our cell membranes that creates the electrical current responsible for nerve impulses. Still, another difference, noted Ashcroft, "between the electrical signals in our heads and in our homes is their speed of transmission. An electrical signal in a wire travels at the speed of light." By comparison, the impulses we generate in our bodies are much slower and smaller in voltage.

We are truly bioelectric beings. Physiologists estimate that about one-third of all the oxygen we take into our lungs and almost half of all the food we consume ends up being used by our bodies to maintain our bio-electrical system or our cell batteries, which are the ion levels of cell membranes.[90] In turn, our nerve fibers, like a superhighway, are responsible for transmitting these electrical signals within our system, with our brain acting as the command center for the entire system. Our brain, heart, nerves, and muscles all generate their own electrical signals, which can be detected by various technological devices. For example, an EEG (electroencephalogram) records brain waves, which constitute voltage changes collectively generated by millions of nerve cells.[91] In animals, this is often manifested as bioluminescence - the biochemical emission of light by living organisms such as fireflies and deep-sea fish.[92] A good example of this is the Atolla Jellyfish. "The Atolla wyvillei jellyfish uses its bioluminescence qualities as a defense mechanism[93]. When in danger, the creature illuminates its organs, specifically its 8 gonads that make up the thick circular ring in the middle of the jellyfish. This creates a very bright blue light that radiates from the scyphozoa. This is used to distract the predator or possibly scare them. Scientists believe that this is used to get the attention of bigger predators to attack the smaller predator hunting the jellyfish. These distracting qualities of the bright blue light give the jellyfish time to evade danger while the larger predator eats the smaller one—not the glowing creature."

Ion Channels are receptacles that network throughout your body allowing subtle energy to interact with every system that makes you a healthy and functional human. Ion channels can also be found in plants, but they function somewhat differently than those in human and animal life. Ashcroft observed, "The electrical impulses of plants differ from those of nerves in that they are of longer duration, travel more slowly, and are carried by different ions," It is well established that in all living things, there is energy that can manifest as light, given the right biological tools. We will examine later in this book the accumulating evidence that these bio-field energies of plants can be harnessed to assist the human bio-field in self-healing and health maintenance.

'Folklore' Validated in Laboratories

Decades ago, I began to question why the most conservative physicians measured the electromagnetic frequency of human organs and body systems using devices like the EKG and EEG, yet the same medical professionals completely ignored these frequencies when it came to their treatment protocols. It was tantamount to scientists measuring the temperature outside without ever examining the effects that temperature can have on forms of life. Looking at all living things as light and vibration that ultimately manifests into energy and matter simplified for me the clarity of how medicine could and should proceed. Many ancient cultures have historically known this truth.

Throughout recorded history, people living in different parts of the world have sensed or intuited the existence of energy fields emanating from humans and other life forms. The ancient Asian healing traditions of Qi Gong and Acupuncture, for instance, evolved from a belief system that viewed the human body as a vehicle of vital energy whose meridians or energy channels can be manipulated to bring about healing and health.

Words such as 'chi' (life force) from China, and 'prana' from India, were expressed several thousand years ago. These terms were created in order to describe this life force energy. Some highly perceptive people reported an ability to see it manifest around the body like a heat haze in the form of colors. We now call these colors 'biofrequency' and have concrete evidence that it radiates from all living things. Biofrequency found in humans extends from head to toe, projecting in layers on average of four feet in all directions. Think of this phenomenon as the visible evidence of the human energy field. The field radiates outward from the body and dynamically changes based on one's physical condition, a person's state of feelings and motivations, and their interactions with the energy radiation projected from other life forms, as well as inanimate objects.

"Things that appear in folklore often turn out to have a basis in fact," observed the surgeon and biofield researcher, Dr. Robert O. Becker.[94] That has certainly been true with biofield research confirmation of observations made over thousands of years.

Humanity's first documented photograph of a biofrequency was credited to the 19th-century electrical scientist and inventor Nikola Tesla. Tesla is known for his contributions to the design of alternating-current electricity. Several decades later, the Russian scientists Seymon and Valentina Kirlian created a method to photograph this energy, which came to be known as Kirlian photography. It involved sending an electric current through an object to capture an image on a photographic plate. The Kirlian image is the phenomenon of allegedly capturing the electrical coronal discharges from an object. [95]

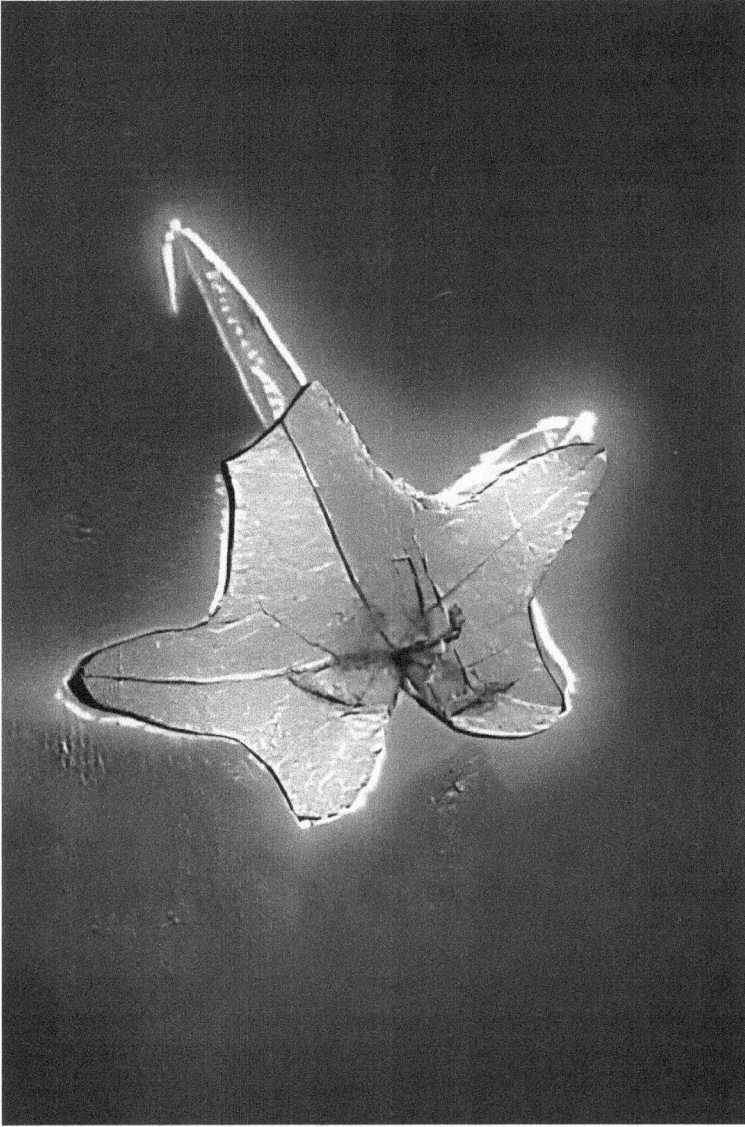

In one noteworthy early experiment, the Kirlians photographed an electrical current sent through two leaves--- one taken from a diseased plant, the other snipped from a healthy plant. They discovered that the image of the healthy leaf appeared bright and luminescent, whereas the unhealthy leaf projected a weak image. There is by no means a consensus on the validity of Kirlian photographs. Many serious and valid doubts exist. Pioneering bio-electric researcher Dr. Becker, author of *The Body Electric: Electromagnetism and the Foundation of Life,* conducted a series of experiments on Kirlian photography during the mid-1970s and found evidence that rather than a biofield being documented, these photos showed corona discharges from the water content of the plant, or from the person. Kirlian halo images were found to remain even after the organism died and "remained the same as long as the water content of the corpse remained constant," noted Becker.

Even with these findings, Becker acknowledged, "This is not to say that the [bio-energy] occasionally perceived by some people around other organisms is imaginary...the [energy] could literally be a form of light, perhaps at frequencies invisible to all but a few of us." He noted how "all living things generate weak electromagnetic fields," and though these biofields are much weaker than the surrounding electromagnetic field of the planet, sensitive people may still perceive them.[96]

In his book *Consciousness Bioenergy and Healing*, Daniel J. Benor, M.D., had this to say about visually perceiving energy fields:

"What seems clear is that a biological energy field exists around the body that is visible to some people, probably more through clairsentient perception than through visual perception. Others can sense such fields with their hands. This ability is much more common than the ability to perceive auras visually. "As with many other aspects of energy medicine, Kirlian phenomena have not been consistently replicable by all investigators, or under all circumstances by the same investigators. This has unfortunately contributed to the rejection of a potentially useful tool for medical diagnosis. It is unclear as yet what Kirlian pictures actually represent. The majority of scientists studying Kirlian photography believe that the image reflects the biological energy state of the subject. If we assume this to be a valid theory, then interactional effects between Kirlian auras of several persons suggest that there are field interactions among living things when they are in close proximity with each other. This suggests a possible basis for how spiritual healing may work. No controlled studies have been published to support this view. Some skeptics think that Kirlian images represent...fluctuations in skin moisture." [97]

Dr. Valerie Virginia Hunt was a distinguished American scientist, author, and a pioneer in bioenergy research. She was the first female professor in the Department of Physiological Sciences at the University of California, Los Angeles (UCLA), where she began her tenure in 1948.

Dr. Hunt's career at UCLA spanned several decades until her retirement in 1980, when she gained recognition for her groundbreaking research on human bioenergy fields and their relationship to health, disease, and emotional pathologies.

Dr. Hunt was renowned for her innovative approach to exploring the human energetic system from a scientific perspective. She was the first scientist to measure the human bioenergy field in a laboratory setting, using high-frequency electronic instruments to record vibrations.

Her work led to the development of the first scientific understanding of how energy field disturbances correlate with physical and emotional conditions. This groundbreaking research culminated in her seminal work, Infinite Mind: Science of the Human Vibrations of Consciousness, published in 1996[98], which provided scientific evidence for individualized energy field signatures and their changes in response to emotional and environmental factors.

Beyond her work in academia, Dr. Hunt served as the Executive Director of the BioEnergy Fields Foundation, a non-profit organization dedicated to advancing research on human bioenergy and applying this knowledge across fields such as medicine, psychology, and education. She also contributed to space biology research for NASA and served as a field reader for U.S. Department of Health, Education, and Welfare research grants. Dr. Hunt's contributions have earned her international acclaim in the fields of physiology, medicine, and bioengineering, bridging the gap between science and holistic health practices.

Valerie Hunt Advances the Research

Research into the human energy field and its projection of visible light was subsequently advanced by a dozen years of high-frequency recordings at Dr. Valerie Hunt's UCLA laboratory. Her experiments began in the early 1970s when one of her graduate students asked for an explanation of what was occurring physiologically when she participated in trance dancing.

Dr. Hunt placed EKG sensors on the student's body. The student danced to trance music as Hunt recorded the muscle tissue and organ frequencies. Data from the electrodes picked up pulses during the dance that seemed to originate from a source other than her physical systems. Dr. Hunt repeated these tests numerous times and realized that she was measuring a dynamic field of energy surrounding the human body that had never been recorded by scientific instruments.

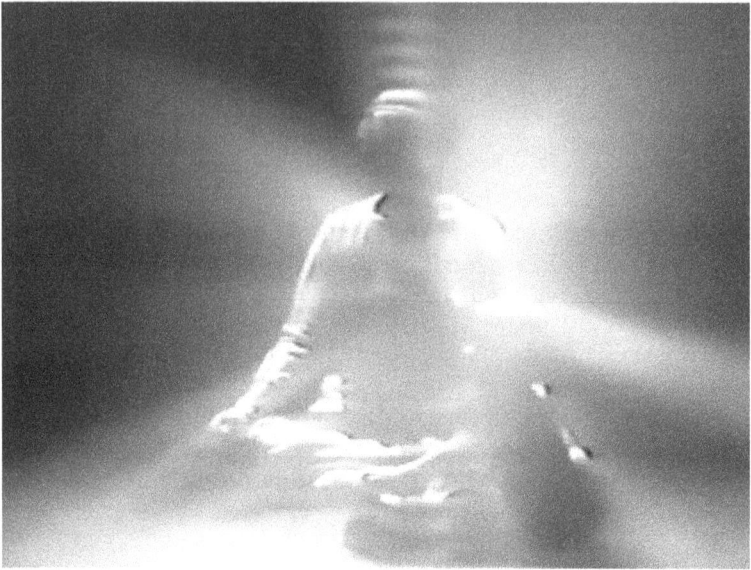

At this stage of the research, her instruments weren't sensitive enough to pick up the full range and intensity of the energy fields. Standard medical devices such as EEG and EKG register only as high as 100 to 150 Hz, and she needed to go far beyond that range. She sought assistance from scientists at NASA who had developed telemetry devices for astronauts to measure their vital signs while on space missions. They helped her create a new research device, an Aura Meter[99], as she called it, a piece of equipment that could measure frequencies up to 250,000 Hz, a thousand times more sensitive than what medical science had in use.

High-frequency energy coming from the surface of the body is picked up by the Aura Meter and computer processing reveals the patterns unique to each individual. These patterns are the biomarkers of disease, behavior, and levels of consciousness. These findings led Dr. Hunt to the study of ritualistic healing, acupuncture and other ancient Asian systems of human body energy mapping. Her goal became to perfect the use of scientific instruments in creating maps of human bio-energy fields in order to show their relationship to human health, behavior, and spirituality.

Dr. Valerie Hunt, UCLA Professor.

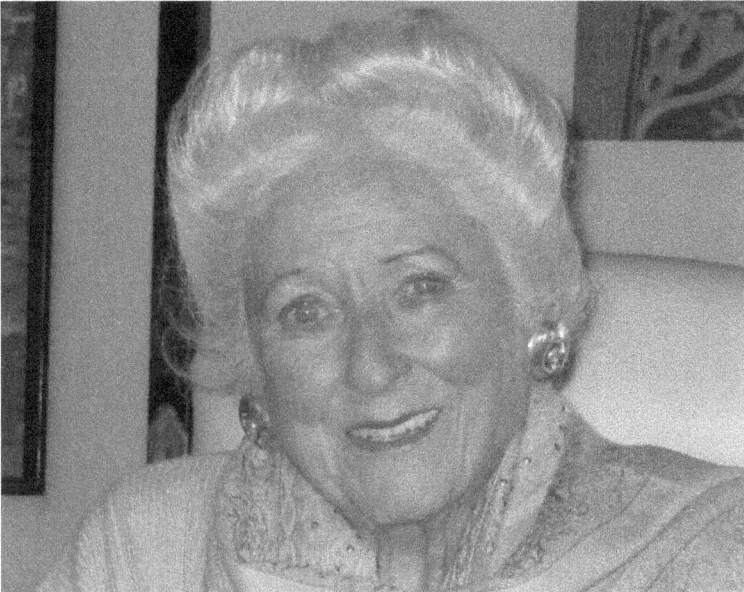

Dr. Hunt stood on the shoulders of a distinguished group of scientific giants in the quantum field, such as:

Harold Saxton Burr, who measured Biological EM fields throughout his work between the years of 1916 and 1956. Burr was a professor at the Yale University Department of Medicine. Using plant seeds, slime molds, trees, amphibians and mammals, he concluded that every living system has a field, and that it can be measured by placing the electrodes on its surface.[100]

Another progressive scientist who offered quantum insight was Daniel J. Benor. He mentions Burr's studies in his book, *Consciousness Bioenergy and Healing*. "These EM (electromagnetic) fields vary over time, and are highly correlated in regular patterns with growth, development, physiological processes, disease, wound healing, and emotional conditions." Benor continues, "Patterns of variation were noted with external factors, such as correlations with atmospheric and earth potentials as well as with lunar cycles and sunspots. Labeling this phenomenon the L-field (life-field), Burr speculated that it provides a template for the maintenance of relative structural and biochemical constancy…he speculated that the L-fields may also function as organizers for growth and development of the organism." Burr's findings echoed that of many physicists, advanced biologists, and even chemists. There was finally a foundation of evidential science that would be the beginning of future medicine.

Leonard Ravitz, an American physician, took Burr's research a step further. He reviewed numerous measurements of electrodynamic states in humans in a wide variety of conditions and found that field perturbations accompanied many physical symptoms.[101] They also correlated with schizophrenia and depression. My work over the last five decades has inherently revealed abnormal frequencies in all psychological and emotional conditions. In such cases we employ biofrequency technologies, clinically observing a taming of many of the symptoms. This is evidence of the electrical component in such disorders.

One individual, Mary, had severe depression from the time she was a child. In her early 20s, this bloomed into manic depression (bipolar disorder). Within a matter of 72 hours, after our medical team applied cold laser and biophoton therapies, her symptoms waned for the first time in forty years. This individual is representative of what we have observed since we began applying electromagnetic therapies in 1980.

Another example was Samuel. He had been diagnosed with a severe form of schizophrenia bordering on multiple-personality disorder. His ability to focus and articulate was minimal. Within ten days after applying subtle frequencies to his brain and nervous system, there was a marked change in his behavior. Not only did he begin to articulate more coherently, but he looked you in the eyes when he spoke. Six months later, it was reported by his psychiatrist that he no longer required meds and was living symptom-free. This disease that Samuel had endured for three decades is not typically arrested in such an abrupt and definitive way. Yet, it is an example of what can be achieved when the right electrical pulses are applied, replenishing the deficiencies in the individual's system.

One of the pillar therapies that we utilize here at Hippocrates is advanced bio-frequency treatments. It is important to note that every individual that we work with is encouraged to adopt a clean, plant-based diet absent of sugars, excessive fats, chemicals and heavy metals. Living food nutrition is that which has not been heated over 115 degrees and vibrates at frequencies that your body's biofrequency system requires.

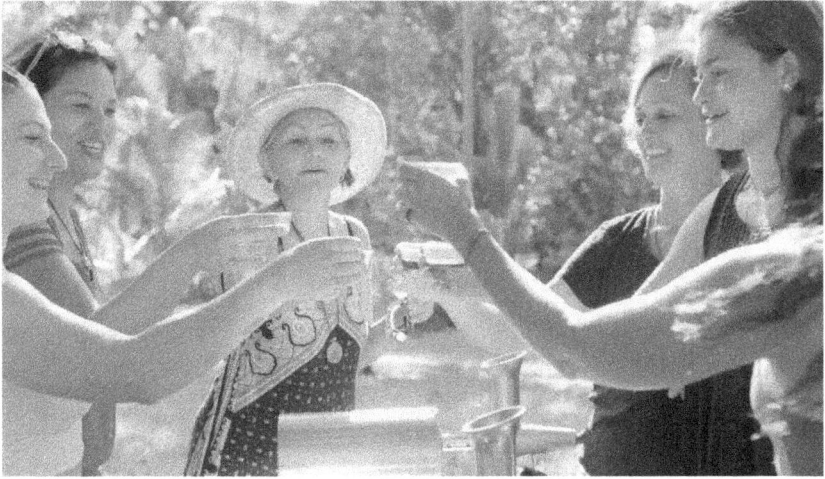

Credits: Wellness: A Journey of Transformation - Hippocrates Wellness Documentary - www.youtube.com/watch?v=5TssMCjZQYM (YouTube)[102]

Dr. Vollert's Bion Therapy

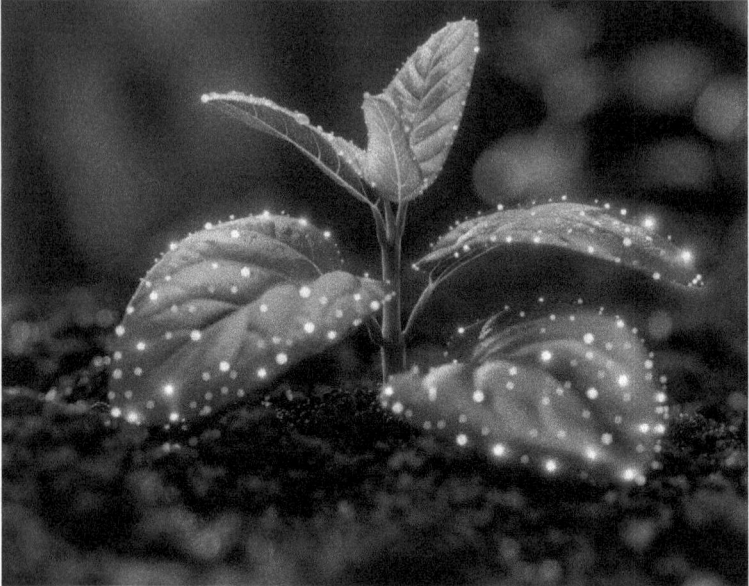

Several years ago, when in Europe, I had the privilege of meeting physician and research professor Dr. Hegall Vollert[103]. We instantly clicked because, over the last six decades, he has worked with what he terms "future medicine." Our professional relationship grew, and I have had him come to the Institute and present to our participants and team. There is no doubt that he is Europe's foremost authority on frequency medicine. His technology has won awards and international acclaim.

He, I, and many others believe that the entire universe, all life, and all atoms are governed by an infinite subtle energy field. All matter is born into existence through the compression of this field. In physical terms, we are talking about standing waves of endless magnitude. All matter is "tuned in" to this field and resonates in unification. This pervading substance is also known as vacuum compression energy (nearly the entire cosmos is a vacuum) and can be monitored on a natural logarithmic line.

As an example, the Aurora Borealis, is a literal manifestation of energy in action.

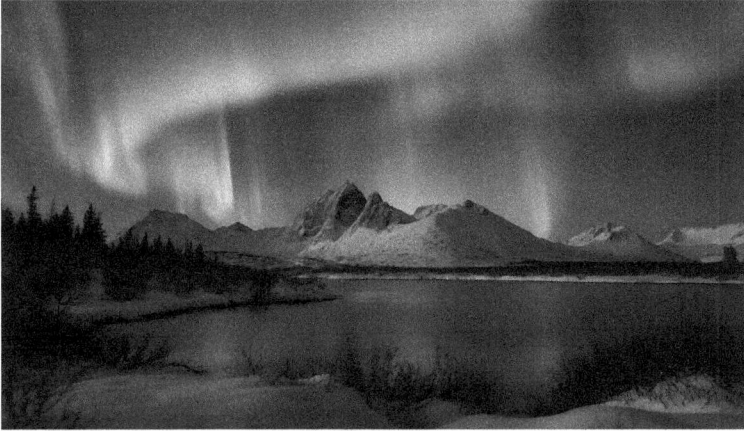

The era of vacuum compression energy and its application in medicine has only just begun. This is in part due to the fact that the chemical aspects of life are overrated and the pulse magnetic aspects underrated. Vacuum compression energy acts as a regulator; it directs the hundreds of thousands of simultaneously occurring metabolic reactions of all cells in all living things. Without this direction, cells would die in seconds due to uncontrolled chemical reactions. In addition, new cells would be unable to form since they would not have the subtle energetic force necessary to welcome them.

The cell acts both to emit and receive energy and information. As a transmission system, it enters a resonant state with various wavelengths from the expansive vacuum compression energy system. These waves pulsate in strict geometric patterns, and according to Vollert, "they represent information and should be considered the principal architect of life and health."

His exploration of this cutting-edge science began as a student when he read the body of work by Wilhelm Reich. Reich's brilliance in the early part of the 20th century, along with his contemporaries like Einstein, Reif, and Tesla, all understood that every organism requires a steady influx of invisible energy in order to maintain a healthy cell structure. Wilhelm's term was 'orgone.'[104]

Below is a chart from Wilhelm Reich, scientifically capturing Orgone in the environment.[105]

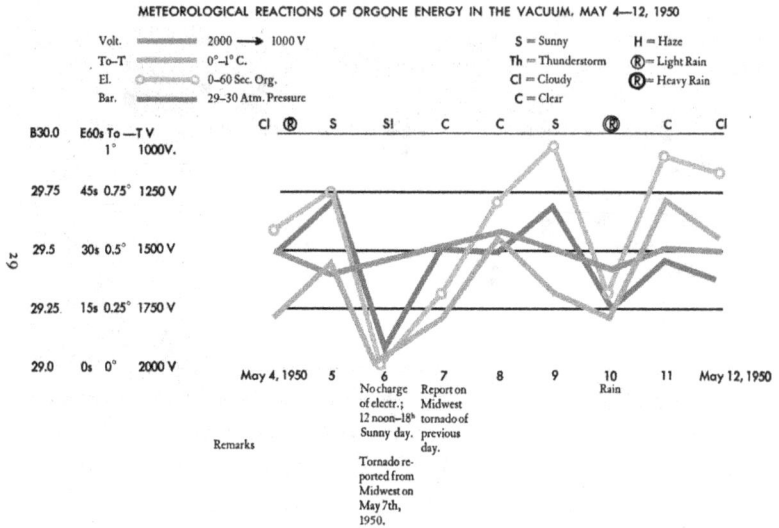

METEOROLOGICAL REACTIONS OF ORGONE ENERGY IN THE VACUUM, MAY 4—12, 1950

Hegall began experimenting with limited knowledge and as time unfolded and he developed a greater understanding, he recognized that there was a way to capture this energy and utilize it in the quest for superior health.

Vollert's Bion therapy works with basic elements that symbiotically manifest a representation of the universal energy. He discovered cloth was a perfect host to harbor this energy. When applying this to parts of the anatomy, it readjusts the body to its normal cellular homeostasis.

Here at Hippocrates Institute, we conducted a double-blind study applying activated and non-activated cloth. Working with more than 100 participants who applied the active and non-active technology, those applying the Bion therapy universally showed measurable changes in their immunity. In addition, 78% of the group using the activated cloth verbally reported feeling better and, in some cases, a noticeable reduction in pain, stress, or discomfort.

Dr. Vollert also designed a calming room that we will build in the future so that our program participants can gain full-body benefits by ingratiating in an environment that mimics the origin of life. The images on the next page show a person's body in its normal state vs after being placed in an unnatural situation. You can see how agitated the biofield is after the body was bombarded with the disruptive and unnatural frequencies from a cellphone. In contrast, captured after the person got themselves in sync with the harmony of nature by touching wheatgrass for one minute, the auras are soothed and calm.

St. Sch. from Sch, m, 22

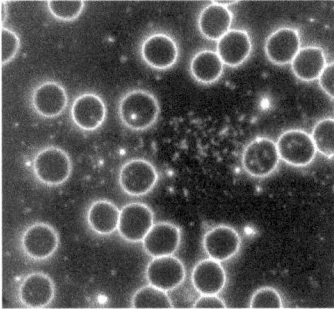

A empty stomach

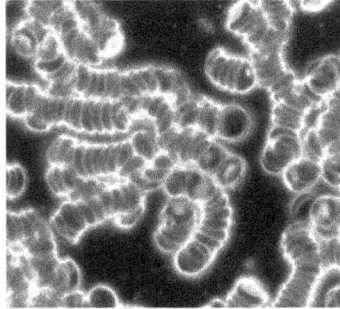

B after 6 min mobile phone call

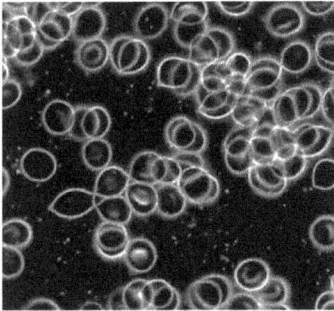

C after 1 min touching wheat grass
(not bion-tec informated)

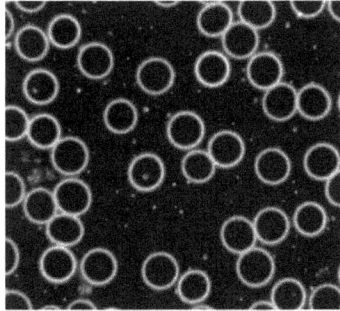

D after 1 min touching wheat grass
(bion-tec informated)

Later, we will be presenting some remarkable work conducted by Hegall in Germany on the growing patterns of seeds and grasses.

Describing Perceived Reality

Torus fields are what alter reality. Sound color and light from scalar waves create TOROIDAL imagery that appears like Op Art, unique geometric patterns that are born out of the frequencies training to audiovisual and invisible waves. These waves permeate all of creation instantly and are always present throughout known space. They move freely and have no definite patterns. They are there for you and all other life to create unique formations from communication going beyond the time/space paradigm.

As far back as 1778, S.J. Brugmans observed what is now known as diamagnetism.[106] Michael Faraday, a scientific showman, displayed this in the mid-19th century with his Faraday cage. His experiments found that some elements and most compounds exhibit a "negative" magnetism. Indeed, all substances are diamagnetic. This field gyrates, speeding up and slowing down the electrons orbiting in atoms in such a way as to oppose the action of the approaching charge particles, repelling their path to approach. Graphite is one visible way that we can see this light magnetic field in action. Magnetite that is in your cells throughout your body also resonates with a charge that permits that cell to keep its form and distance from other cells while in the process of creating your anatomy.

Another part of this story is paramagnetism[107]. This is weaker than general magnetism and is affected by temperature. Oxygen contains a paramagnetic field. Without visibly observing this, ancients in Central Asia correctly hypothesized and stated that when you breathe in, oxygen carries a charge that enhances your well-being and lifts your consciousness so that you can connect to the omnipresent external energies that we now know make up the endless multiple universes.

Today's Quantum science has become so advanced that we can identify that light, color, and sound project outwards and change the universe, which is TOROIDAL itself, but perpetually willing to change its patterns via your contribution.

Language - Energetic Characteristic

Listed below are some vowels that create certain patterns

- **E** = Emotion / Renewal / Change / Transformation
- **O** = Wholeness
- **U** = Restriction
- **I** = Intensity

Previously, language experts at best spoke about words and the effect that they may have on your and other's emotions. At the same time, the loudness, intensity, volume, and presentation were all considered important in terms of what the verbiage personified. Today, we are actually saying that the sound of vowels creates specific patterns, no matter who is verbalizing them, that change the universe and the immediate environment around you and those in your presence.[108] Collective consciousness or collective awareness, otherwise referred to as the tipping point, now has hardcore science validity.[109] To demonstrate that you and those in your presence as well as the endless connectivity to all things and all else is changed when massive communication with the same intention occurs with a large number of people.

Every verbal / emotional contribution we submit adds to the universal fabric and enlists us as an active player in the perpetual cosmic symphony. In addition, the words we choose with the intentions they convey and the vibration released into the world through speech have the ability to shape our individual lives and that of collective awareness.

One proven and successful therapy that helps to readjust your neuron functions is neurolinguistic therapy.[110] This thoughtful contribution to personal evolution teaches us to observe and listen to the words we choose and ultimately becoming more purposeful in our communication. Choirs throughout history that honor the internal and external spirit have done so in the homage of elevated comprehension.

Food Frequency

As Dr. Robert Archer expresses in his thesis, there are five phases of energetics in food.

- **Enzymes** - Lifeforce in organic raw life plants
- **Micro-biotics** - Comprehensively embrace plant energy
- **Prebiotics-** The enzyme-rich cellulose in green plants that feed gut bacteria in the production of immune system cells
- **Probiotics -** The living bacteria within the cells of edible plants that feed vital serotonin brain function
- **Biofrequency field -** Universal network that all life forms contain

Each of these magnificent energies and frequency-producing vibrations are active messengers from the plant kingdom to we homo sapiens. An ongoing conversation occurs when you embrace vibrant, unfired living food that enhances your ability to open your imagination, improve your verbal expression, and deeply comprehend your purpose.

CHAPTER 7:

We Are All 'Light' Beings

"If you want to find the secrets of the universe, think in terms of energy, frequency, and vibration. - Nikola Tesla (1856-1943) Serbian-American inventor, engineer and physicist

Every living thing constantly absorbs and transmits light[111]. In the case of humans, this light transmission occurs from numerous points on the body, particularly from the fingers and the palms of our hands, though this light is invisible to the unaided eye. Using a powerful photon counter device, a team of photonic scientists in Japan measured these light emissions in 2005 and found that all humans release streams of weak photons through their fingernails, fingers, and palms of the hands. The highest light emission levels of the study volunteers were found to be from the fingers and fingernails, though other weak photon emissions were discovered to come from the forehead and the bottoms of both feet. These findings were reported in *the Journal of Photochemistry and Photobiology.*

Since then, hundreds of studies have been conducted examining many aspects of how and why bio photons are emitted from the human frame. Clear distinctions were found between these light emissions and the other invisible form of light, infrared radiation, that emanates from body heat.

For instance, in 2009, another team of Japanese scientists, from Kyoto University, found that, in their words, "the human body literally glimmers.[112] We found that the human body directly and rhythmically emits light. This energy is released as light through the changes in energy metabolism." A daily rhythm of photon emission was detected in the bodies of volunteers, usually peaking in the late afternoon, as cortisol levels in the body decreased during the same period. "Our findings suggest that cameras that can spot the weak emissions could help spot medical conditions," commented Hitoshi Okamura, a circadian biologist and co-author of the report.[113] A clue as to how spotting medical conditions using biophotons could happen and be perfected came in a study published in the *Journal of Experimental Biology*, which examined biophoton emissions from normal skin cells and cancerous (melanoma) skin cells. Scientists found that "remarkable differences between normal and cancer cells" could be distinguished based on their photon emissions as detected by a UVA laser. "In this respect," the scientists wrote, "this powerful and noninvasive technique can be applied in a variety of skin research, such as the investigation of skin abnormalities and to test the effect of treatments involved in regeneration and remedies for progressive medicine."[114] A team of researchers in Germany at The International Institute of Biophysics discovered this correlation between a person's health and the level of photon emissions from their body.[115] The weaker their immune system, the weaker and more erratic the emissions of light. One of the world's leading scientific authorities on biological photon emissions, German physicist Fritz-Albert Popp, noted how these studies replicated some of his own findings from the 1970s, that further showed a correlation between a person's health and their projection of light. Being a manifestation of life's light reflected in anatomical structure. We can heal ourselves with appropriate living plant nutrition. Light and laser treatment will be employed in future medicine.

Herbs and Mind Power Affect Light Transmission

An additional realm of research that could revolutionize healthcare and health diagnostics involves the impact of the human mind on biophoton emissions. Biophotons are photons of light in the ultraviolet spectrum and low visible light range that are produced by a biological system. Medical dictionaries define biophoton emissions as low energy endogenous radiation produced by humans and other living organisms and detected as a barely visible light.

There is a natural level of photon emission, which is released when the parasympathetic nervous system is engaged. As a bulb on the end of a wire, our biological light grows brighter when it resonates with particular healing frequencies. Certain foods and positive thoughts carry these healing frequencies, providing support for the immune system. On the other hand, when "food" or sluggish or excessive frequencies enter our bodies that do not resonate appropriately, they can cause immune system degradation. In these instances, the light is too dim, or frequencies overwhelm the bulb, causing it to fail.

Research has documented how ingesting certain herbs and engaging in meditation practice both influence a person's biophoton output. Using the herbal supplement Rhodiola rosea, known for its cortisol and stress reduction powers, scientists in The Netherlands tested 30 lab volunteers against a control (placebo) group. In the week before and after supplementation, photon emissions were measured, using a biophoton counter device on the dorsal side of the participant's hands. Stress and fatigue levels were also measured. Compared to the control group, those taking Rhodiola showed a "significant decrease" in photon emission, along with a "significant decrease" in stress and fatigue.[116] Measuring the impact of an herb on human biophoton emissions needs to be expanded to include a wide range of nutrients. When assessed using this biophoton counter device, which charts positive and negative influences at the cellular level, both the health-rejuvenating nutrients of raw living foods and the health-depleting toxins of junk foods and animal products impact the human body.

German and Dutch scientists studied the biophoton emissions from a group of 20 volunteers (20 to 65 years of age), half of whom were experienced meditators using the TM practice. They studied both groups, who were placed in a dark room and had their biophoton emissions measured from 12 body regions, extending from their head and torso to their hands. Biophoton emissions were found to be, overall, 35% lower in the meditators compared to the non-meditators. This biophoton reduction was true in all body areas except the palms of their hands, where both groups showed similar emission levels. The researchers speculated that the lower biophoton emission levels in meditators was a phenomenon due to them having lower levels of stress because "stress is connected to increased production of reactive oxygen species and related chemical reactions resulting in cell and tissue damage."[117] Still, another important science study showing the mind's impact on biophoton emission was published in the journal *Neuroscience Letters* in 2012. Canadian scientists discovered that when volunteers *imagined light* while they were inside a completely dark room, they created "significant increases" in the biophoton emissions being measured from the right sides of their heads. The research team's conclusion was that "specific visual imagery is strongly correlated with ultra-weak photon emission coupled to brain activity."[118]

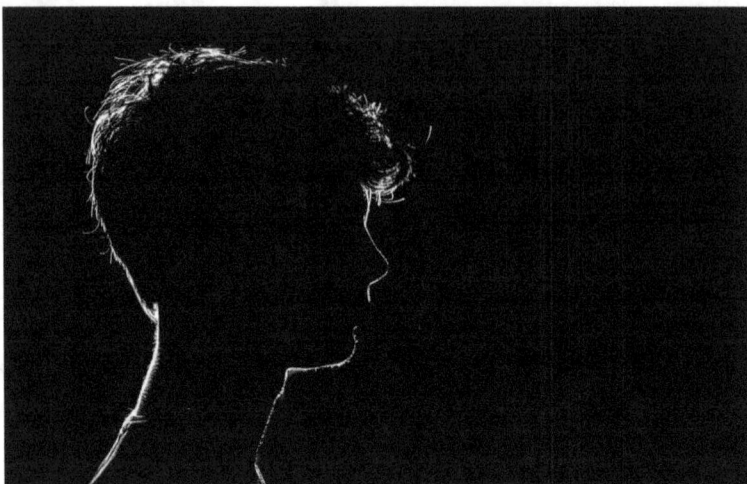

To identify which part of the brain is most directly correlated to biophoton emissions, scientists writing in *NeuroQuantology, An Interdisciplinary Journal of Neuroscience and Quantum Physics*, described how they used volunteers to measure photon emissions and brain waves (EEG) simultaneously. "The data suggest significant correlations between fluctuations in photon emission and fluctuations in the strength of alpha wave production in the 7-13 Hz frequency band and its 1-Hz sub-bands." This data was found to be "in relationship to mind-body interactions and the role of consciousness in health."[119]

Alpha brain waves (8-12 Hz) usually occur when you are daydreaming or engaging in meditation or mindfulness practices.[120] Other synchronized electrical activity, or brain waves, are Beta, when attention is focused on tasks, and Gamma, when information is quickly being processed.

Brain scientists writing in the science journal *Cortex* found the first conclusive evidence in 2015 that "specifically enhancing alpha oscillations is a causal trigger of creativity." This effect also reduced depression. Non-invasive brain stimulation, in 20 volunteer test subjects using a transcranial alternating current, detected frontal brain areas being activated, producing alpha waves, which, in turn, triggered creativity as measured by tests of creative thinking.[121]

This link between brain alpha waves, heightened biophoton emissions, and increased creativity is a fertile area for further research to determine how 'hands-on' healing may be consciously activated and energy transferred during healing sessions.

Brain Wave Technology for Stress Relief

NuCalm is an innovation that manipulates the brain's alpha waves. It is utilized at the Hippocrates Institute, which I direct, to quickly induce deep states of calm and relaxation.

It entails a process with four components: First, you apply either a NuCalm topical cream, or chew dietary supplements which utilize neurotransmitter nutrients to counteract adrenaline in the body. Then, microcurrent stimulation patches are placed behind each of the ears. Noise-dampening headphones are worn, through which neuroacoustic software delivers a low electrical current frequency to bring brain waves to a pre-sleep stage of alpha and theta ranges. Eye masks are worn to block out ambient light.

This technology has proven useful for dentists and doctors to calm patients before surgical procedures and prescribed for patients who have difficulty getting deep, quality sleep. It's also beneficial for patients whose bodies can't tolerate drugs given for sedation. Athletes use it before competition to manage cortisol release and for faster recovery from injuries.

NuCalm was originally designed by a neuroscientist to treat post-traumatic stress disorder.[122] Many of the world's leaders, including Anthony Robbins, and many star athletes on sports teams globally, use it as rejuvenation therapy, particularly in the face of their demanding travel schedules.

Brain Tap is another technology that employs ten sensory stimulators that were formulated by a physician who also has an advanced understanding of electronics. Mapping out the regions of the brain that provoke certain reactions allowed him to target it so the desired results can be accomplished. Be it relaxation, contemplation, sleep, or immune stimulation. We are now forging a new frontier of helping to remove either blocked energy, excessive energy, or the dissolution of weak energy. Applying this technology in a clinical setting has further revealed the absolute control of biological functions via brain/thought activity. One perfect example is that when utilizing Brain Tap, it is evident that it turns on 2300 positive gene expressions. This by the way, can alter and improve one's state of health, lifespan, extending longevity.

The Power of Hands-On-Healers

Healers channel light through their hands. Light pulsing from the human body becomes irregular in people with weakened immune systems, illnesses or disease. Consequently, biological light projected into those who are enduring illness by hands-on healers during healing sessions seems to power up the recipient's healing cells.

These observations lend support to an even more intriguing pair of laboratory discoveries. When bio-energy healers, using techniques called Reiki and Therapeutic Touch, are engaged in their healing practices, surges of both light and electrostatic charges have been recorded as emerging from their hands for periods ranging from one to twelve seconds in duration, with a voltage range from 4 to 221 volts at a time.

A lab study at the Columbus Polarity Therapy Institute in Columbus, Ohio, found "consistent and dramatic" fluctuations in the gamma rays (high-frequency electromagnetic fields) throughout the bodies of all ten test subjects receiving hands-on healing.[123] These anomalous alterations in electromagnetic fields provide some of the strongest evidence yet for the healing force of nature being harnessed by focus and intentional practices. In these studies, the human body was used as a conductor to activate cellular and molecular processes that may be beneficial to healing. All of us possess this inherent frequency. We can exercise it and properly employ it to serve the healing process.

At the University Of Miami School Of Medicine, researchers with the Touch Research Institute have been documenting the medical benefits of human touch through a series of studies published in peer-reviewed journals.

Among the study findings:

- **Immune system** - The function is heightened by human touch. Natural killer cells showed increased activity in women with breast cancer and HIV patients.

- **Pain reduction** - Cortisol levels were lowered and pain intensity decreased in children with mild to moderate juvenile rheumatoid arthritis after touch therapy.

- **Mental performance and alertness** - Human touch has been shown to sharply enhance adult cognitive abilities.

Touch is an energy exchange. As Tiffany Field, PhD, director of the Touch Research Institute, pointed out, touching is good for both the facilitator and the recipient. Her studies have demonstrated that senior citizens decrease their stress hormone levels and need fewer doctor visits after giving massages to infants.

Similarly, when the parents of children with leukemia gave daily massages to their kids, the parents experienced greater mental and physical health, and their children showed increased white blood cell counts. (For summaries of these and dozens of other 'touch power' studies by Field and colleagues, go to: **www6.miami.edu/touch-research/ChildMassage.html.**)

"While Western medicine has focused primarily on the physical body, Progressive Medicine therapists have long been aware that living creatures also possess biological energy bodies—which are composed of emotional, mental, relational, and spiritual levels of subtle pulses.... Each of these biofield levels is intimately interlinked with the others. Each level contributes to our states of health and illness, and each energy field may be addressed, individually, or in concert with the others, to improve physical, psychological, relational and spiritual health." - Daniel J. Benor, M.D., in his book, *Consciousness Bioenergy and Healing.*

Numerous complementary treatments affect the human body's biological energies, ranging from Therapeutic Touch and Reiki, to traditional Chinese medicine, Biofrequency Technology Medicine, Acupuncture, Homeopathy, and Naturopathic Medicine. These subtle energies include electrical and magnetic effects and some emitting forces that have been measured but otherwise remain unidentified or labeled. Spontaneous remissions are one byproduct of the manipulation of these subtle energies either by a practitioner or from the mental processes initiated by the patient.

Yet another team of Japanese scientists found that strong biomagnetic fields could be measured around the hands of a wide range of healing and martial arts experts in such disciplines as meditation, Qigong, and Yoga. The fields they measured showed up to 0.0010 gauss, or about 1,000 times more intense than the cardiac (heart) field, previously thought to be the strongest field in the human body.[124] Many ancients were aware of these human healing energies. The Chinese utilized them through practices like Tai Chi and Qigong. Hippocrates understood human-energy power as well. He said, "The natural healing force within each of us is the greatest force in getting well."

The Constant Rhythm of our Energy Fields

Our heart and brain both generate electromagnetic fields[125], and every cell in our body acts as an antenna/receiver for these signals. These energy fields project outwards and can be detected by sensitive instruments. Other invisible fields of energy, including nuclear, gravitational, and magnetic, surround us, and their signals, including radio and television, pass through our bodies every second. Our bodies are organized energy systems interconnected by energy fields that radiate beyond our bodies at the speed of light into space and interact with other types of energy fields, including the subtle fields projected by other humans.

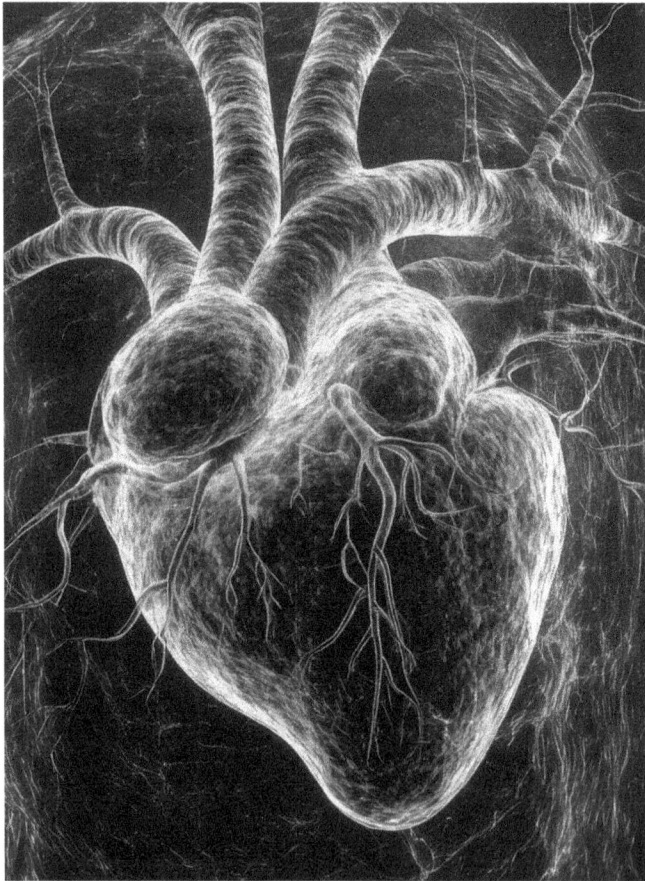

Our Hands Act as Antenna Projecting Bio-Field Energy

Up until just a couple of years ago, mainstream scientists and physicians scoffed at the idea that human beings emit detectable levels of light. Religious figures have long made this claim, and in the last few decades, cutting-edge researchers investigating energy healing have also made it.

Since 2006, a series of lab experiments from prestigious research institutes have documented and confirmed that humans emit measurable levels of light from their hands, and healers engaged in 'hands-on' healing sessions project and amplify much higher levels than ordinary people.[126] "We now know that light is a major component of the vibratory communication system of the body, because such vibrations have been both predicted on the basis of fundamental biophysical theory, and measured by sensitive devices," observed James Oschman, PhD., writing in his book, *Energy Medicine in Therapeutics and Human Performance.* "The role of light in living processes has passed from the 'hallucination' stage to current science." The latest findings on the sciences of light are recorded in a technical periodical entitled *Biophotonics International.*

"There exists a relationship which is largely predictable between light frequency, environment, and the restoration of health following departures from the normal, which are still within the physiologic limits," said Dr. H.R. Spitler, quoted in Oschman's book. Oschman continued: "Dr. Spitler's observation that, within limits, health can be restored with specific light frequencies poses a profound biological question: How can light 'jump start' the healing process for a wide range of clinical problems involving tissue throughout the body?"

An article in the *Journal of Optometric Phototherapy* rephrased the question this way: "How does light find the right places to work to heal the body? Normal tissue is much less affected by light than out-of-balance tissue. Starving cells are far more sensitive than well-fed ones."[127] Light, being the source of all life, infuses its subtle yet powerful energy into weak and injured cells. Cell death (apoptosis) is greatly reduced when the frequency of an energetic fix is afforded to diseased tissue.

Dispelling Medical Science Dogma

Regeneration has been genetically programmed into us; every second we live, we regenerate cells in our body. After about seven years, our bodies have been completely reconstructed at the cellular level. For this reason alone, spontaneous or radical regeneration cannot be dismissed as foreign to our potential or even to our experience.

One theme for this book is how our emotions, our hopes and fears, communicate with our immune system to produce healing molecules and how our bodily electrical system interplays with it. Many ancient doctors, like Hippocrates, taught that if we could remove our emotional blockages, we will be on the path to wellness.

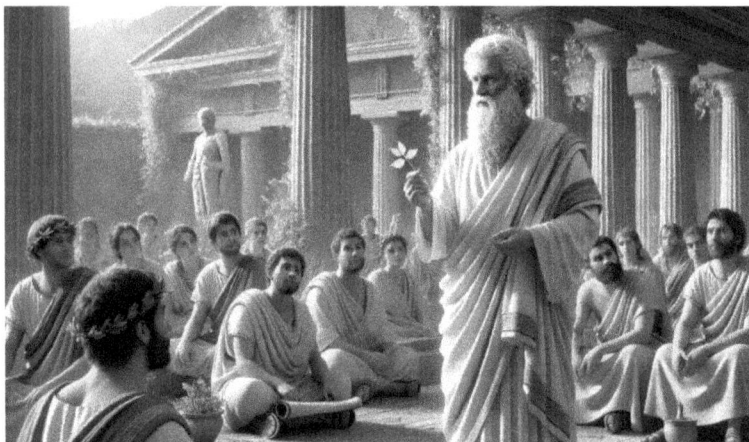

Up until the 1980s, the idea that the human brain could have a direct influence on the immune system was considered laughable by mainstream medical science. In the 1980s, the neuroscientist Dr. David Felten and his research colleagues made a monumental discovery. Under a microscope, they found that nerve fibers extend into every organ where immune cells were present.[128] A new field of psychoneuroimmunology was born, and Felten was at the forefront of revealing the mind's ability to influence the immune system positively. Many of his students embraced his findings, internalizing them and presenting them in their own fashion; one such practitioner was Dr. Brugh Joy.

While attending one of Dr. Brugh Joy's healing energy workshops in the California desert, Michael Crichton, author of *Jurassic Park* and numerous other popular books and movies, had an experience with biofields that astounded him. Crichton earned his medical degree from Harvard Medical

School and showed himself to be an astute observer of medical science and human nature. In his nonfiction book, *Travels*[129], he described how he discovered the reality of human energy fields at this Brugh Joy workshop.

"There isn't any delusion,...It is absolutely clear that this body energy is a genuine phenomenon of some kind. You didn't have to be in the mood to feel it, you didn't have to be a meditating saint, you didn't have to believe in it. You just had to calm down and then hold your hand out over somebody's body, In fact, the body energy was so clearly genuine, so stable and straightforward, that the most common reaction of people in our group was 'Why hasn't anybody told us about this before?" - Dr. Michael Crichton

One of the other medical practitioners participating in the same workshop with Crichton was Dr. Judith Orloff, a Los Angeles psychiatrist who came away equally impressed with the bio-energy transmission demonstrations. Dr. Orloff is an Assistant Clinical Professor of Psychiatry at UCLA, who subsequently held workshops and wrote several books, including, *Guide to Intuitive Healing*[130] and *Positive Energy*, in which she developed the idea that bio-energy could be manipulated to benefit anyone's physical or mental health.

Toward the end of his own 1988 book, Crichton summarized what his direct experience in the bio-energy workshop had taught him;

"There are energies associated with the human body that are not yet understood. These energies can be felt and seen, and they are related to healing, sickness, and health. Although the existence of these body energies is formally accepted in some theoretical systems, such as those of Indian Yogis and Chinese acupuncturists, they are not yet established in Western medical systems. I suspect they will be in the near future."

That 'near future' Crichton referred to is NOW: We are just beginning to understand what Confucius stated a millennium ago: "Knowing what is known, and not knowing what is not known. This is true knowledge." *What is scientifically known today is that your inner photonic energy (soul) is who you are, with the biblically referred to vessel, the body, being a temporary vehicle in the perpetual stream of existence that unifies us to all.* We are on the verge of truly understanding the power within us. Through this knowledge of self and self-belief, we can immediately engage. All of us can be well educated on this phenomenon to tap into our internal energies and heal ourselves.

CHAPTER 8:

Light Treatment Gains Acceptance

Despite its remarkable effectiveness, safety profile, and affordability, light therapy remains for the most part, underappreciated and underused. – Len Saputo, M.D.

At the Center for Light Treatment and Biological Rhythms, affiliated with Columbia University Medical Center in New York, patients with various psychological and mood disorders are routinely prescribed light boxes as a treatment. These sessions of bright light exposure therapy fall under a treatment category known as chronotherapeutics[131], which is timed light exposure to resynchronize the body's biological clock (circadian rhythm) to treat mood, energy, and sleep disorders.

Light therapy has been utilized for years. As clinical experiments of light therapy have expanded, so have the conditions that exposure to light helps alleviate. Everything from chronic fatigue to Alzheimer's disease has been found to be responsive.

"Light is an active pharmacological agent activating the brain," observed Anna Wirz-Justice, a professor at the Psychiatric Hospital of the University of Basel in Switzerland. It works quickly and without side effects. How it produces these results, however, remains a medical mystery.

The best explanation scientists like Professor Wirz-Justice can offer is that bright light exposure jumpstarts sluggish circadian clocks in the human body to bring about therapeutic effects. Dr. Liberman in his book "Light: Medicine of the Future"[132] describes the anatomical workings of photons engaging neurons in the brain. Although this is not taught in the corridors of mainstream medicine, it resonates since the outcomes of employing light in the correction of emotional and biological diseases, have been definitively proven.

A study published in the 2011 *Archives of General Psychiatry*[133], uncovered evidence that light perception and absorption decline with age, so elderly patients might benefit most from light therapy in a variety of ways. The patients in this study received an hour of 7,500 lux pale blue light exposure each morning for three weeks, and every participant experienced greatly improved sleep and enhanced moods. What these developments sketch for us is how we are just beginning to test the boundaries of a proposition that certain wavelengths of light exert profound healing effects.

Many appliance shops in Northern Europe, where sunlight is scarce in the winter months, have long offered full-spectrum lighting boxes that people can use. These are meant to employ to ward off seasonal depression. There are volumes of research studies highlighting the effectiveness of such therapy, yet mainstream physicians tend to treat this disorder with antidepressants.

Since 1999, Dr. Len Saputo[134], an internal medicine specialist affiliated with the John Muir Medical Center in the San Francisco Bay area, has used light therapy to treat more than 2,000 of his patients for a variety of painful health conditions, including neuropathy, neck and back pain, sports injuries, fractures, and even chronic headaches.[135]

In a November 2015 report, Dr. Saputo described the treatment and subsequent recovery of three patients with severe neuropathy (damage or disruption of nerves in the peripheral nervous system, causing loss of sensation, or intense pain) who were given light therapy.

Neuropathies can be caused by diabetes, traumatic injuries, metabolic disorders, or infections. The following three neuropathy patients were documented: Patient Number One was a 69-year-old woman who suffered from advanced peripheral neuropathy, and progressive numbness in her hands and feet, resulting from chemotherapy for colon cancer. She was unable to button her clothing or drive her car.

After 11 light treatments of 15 minutes each, she was able to function at near-normal levels again. In the case of the second patient, a 39-year-old woman, she had been injured in a tornado when a tree crashed around her.

Afterward, she was unable to raise her arms above her head, had lost feeling in her feet and lower legs, and also developed lumbar disc disease. After 7 light therapy treatments, she reported: "Photonic stimulation has been a miracle for me. I no longer have pain when I stand or walk."

With patient number three, a 56-year-old man, health conditions included type 2 diabetes, hypertension, and hyperlipidemia, along with peripheral neuropathy, causing him to take numerous prescription medications. He received 31 infrared light treatments and as a result, he became pain-free and eventually was able to discontinue all of his medications.

Thousands of medical studies over the past few decades have examined the beneficial effects of light therapy treatments for a range of medical conditions: pain, circulation problems, fractures, inflammation, wounds, lymphatic drainage, and much more.

Here are just a few examples cited from various studies:

- **Skin wound repair.** When low-level laser light therapy was applied to both young and aged animals in a lab experiment it was shown to be "an effective treatment of skin wounds" at all stages of the tissue repair process.[138]

- **Skeletal muscle repair.** Seventeen studies were evaluated that had examined low-level laser therapy and its effects on skeletal muscle injuries. Overall findings supported "the positive effects of this therapy on the muscle repair process, the modulation of growth factors, and increased angiogenesis." This technique "is an excellent therapeutic resource."[39]

- **Joint inflammation treatment.** Such inflammation plays a role in the development of osteoarthritis. In this animal lab study, low-level laser therapy (LLLT) operating at 50 mW was found to be effective in reducing joint inflammation and bringing about cellular healing. [140]

Beyond the phenomenal results of using photon (light) therapy, subtle frequencies created at a minuscule level also render impressive results. There is ample evidence that bio-energy in the form of pulsed electromagnetic fields accelerates nerve damage recovery and can regenerate nerves.[136]

Pulsed weak electromagnetic fields have also been shown in lab tests to alleviate symptoms in multiple sclerosis patients, along with the treatment of osteoarthritic joints, pain in post-polio patients, and the mending of broken bones. Though the mechanism is still debated, the effect mirrors and supports the idea of a "human energy field" that is responsive to magnetic influences. The U.S. National Institute of Health, Office of Alternative Medicine, now defines a 'bio-field' as "a massless field, not necessarily electromagnetic, that surrounds and permeates living bodies." Energy fields surrounding human bodies is accepted knowledge.[137] Two researchers at the HeartMath Institute in California, a medical research facility dedicated to the study of the human heart, discovered in 1995 that distant bio-frequency experts could alter the rate of the winding and unwinding of DNA strands in test tubes, a finding that may help to explain a mechanism for radical regeneration since DNA controls many body cell functions.

HeartMath scientists have mastered the new scientific parameters that lead us to better understand the connection between frequencies, pulses, electrons, and human anatomy. Another good example of such data is Dr. Stone's physical touch work that he called "Polarity Therapy."[138]

Gamma radiation (another moniker for bio-energy) technologies have been used to measure the efficacy of Polarity Therapy treatments. In a study of 30 volunteers, anomalous gamma rays were found around the bodies of 100 percent of these test subjects and at every point of their frame. This was achieved using technologies to measure such phenomena.

Polarity therapy works with the natural energy meridians in the human body. Its treatment intends to restore a balanced distribution of body energy. Most bio-frequency experts use the concept of 'energy' as a metaphor, much as one might use the word 'love' to describe a general feeling state. They do not believe the energy or force of nature that they project to be their own. They feel like they channel, or act as a kind of lightning rod, to amplify the energies absorbed from the environment or from an omnipresent multi-universal force, often referred to as zero-point gravity.

Energy Practitioners Alter Magnetic Fields Through Their Hands

These individuals emit frequencies almost identical to the ones measured in healers who use Reiki and other similar techniques. Qigong masters, for example, project strong bio-magnetic fields, an effect first measured in 1992 by scientists in Japan. M.L. Pall's Electromagnetic Fields study from 2013 confirmed, oscillating magnetic fields are known to have effects on neurons, cancer cells, and most organs of the body.[139]

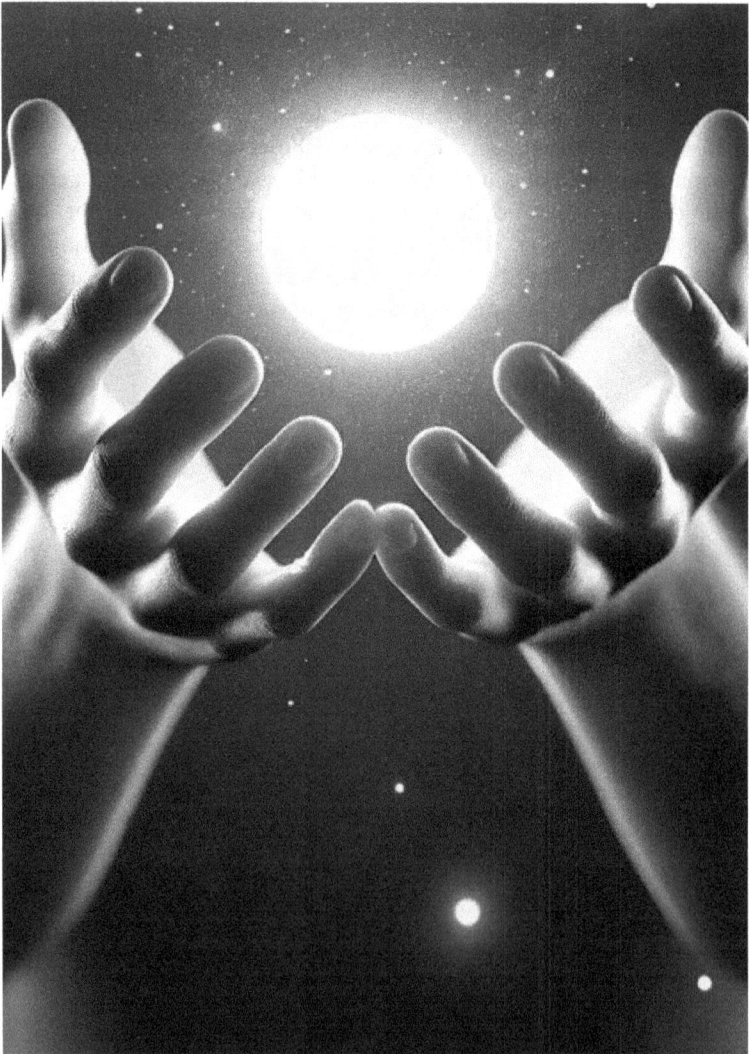

CHAPTER 9:

The Healing Power of Subtle Energy Medicine

It is possible that there exist human emanations which are still unknown to us. Do you remember how electrical currents and 'unseen waves' were laughed at? The knowledge about man is still in its infancy. – Albert Einstein

We know that the sun's rays are the source of life on Earth. All life is generated by light that manifests frequencies. These frequencies are captured and converted into energy. Single-cell life forms and the green plants they spawned possess receptor-like chargeable batteries that convert this energy into matter. Matter has evolved into endless life forms perpetually connected to and containing these frequencies. Energy is the movement of subatomic particles. These subatomic particles are representative of protonic energy that was generated by the sun itself. Depending upon how rapidly they pulsate determines what structure they create. Solid matter is an illusion and just a gathering of these atoms that manifest molecules that become all we see, touch, know, understand, and are.

Dr. Valerie Hunt's research has created what amounts to a new model for the nature of living beings. In this model, all disease is derived from 'anti-coherent' patterns in the human bio-energy field. These anti-coherent patterns spring from the way humans choose to organize their emotional experiences.

"Signature Field" is the term Dr. Hunt applied to each person's unique resting pattern of frequencies. A healthy human being's Signature Field shows coherent and balanced energy patterns across the full spectrum of frequencies.[140]

On a graph, this coherency appears as smooth, gentle, shallow waves that are evenly distributed throughout the frequency spectrum.

By contrast, the Signature Fields of people who have developed or will soon develop various diseases manifest either a deficiency pattern in their energy frequencies (where Qi or energy is lacking) or a hyperactive pattern (where there is too much chi or energy). Both of these abnormal patterns appear on the measurement graph as thick, jagged waves concentrated in high—or low-frequency bands.

Dr. Hunt's research findings further demonstrated that 'deficiency' diseases, like most cancers, produce anti-coherent patterns mostly in the high-frequency range, whereas 'hyperactive' maladies (defined as having faster-moving parts) those caused by microbes, allergies, and some forms of cancer like leukemia, hypertension, and colitis produce patterns entirely in the low-frequency ranges.

Things resonating at low frequencies move quickly, and high frequencies move slowly. Meter readings can identify whether the disease is due to deficiency or hyperactive frequencies[141], though the device cannot specifically identify the organs or tissues that will be attacked.

Contrary to our current understanding of molecular science, less structure allows minute energy to connect with the greater energy field, causing it to pulsate at a higher degree. More mass or structure slows down the rhythmic pulsations. Hunt was excessively successful in assisting many progressive medical physicians in diagnosing diseases that were otherwise undetectable by conventional means.

While genetic and other factors help to determine the target organs and tissues of the body, there is a distinct diagnostic and treatment advantage in having a device like the Aura Meter, able to predict what type of disease will likely occur in advance of the symptoms.

Professor Hunt also used surface skin electrodes to record high-frequency electromagnetic activity under special circumstances: during meditation, emotional states, pain, laying-on-hands healing, and during imaging.[142] She discovered that the patterns in EMG recordings, previously assumed to represent only 'noise,' carry a large amount of information about the person being monitored.

Although genetics is now leading the way into a dynamic improvement of our understanding of human being's totality [143] (consciousness, anatomy, universal connectivity), it will ultimately be found that the mathematics of the unique genetic makeup is a gathering of personalized frequencies that have been captured throughout time in the essential process of making you and all other living things what they are.

Currently at Hippocrates Health Institute, we are using a state-of-the-art heart rate variability and a Russian-made Energy Frequency Biofeedback unit to study biological states and trends in our guests. You will learn more about this in a later chapter.

Conventional Western medicine has concentrated on treating the symptoms of illness and disease. It is a symptom-response frame of mind; a 'take this pill and you will be better' mentality that is a dead end.

When a new drug is first released, there may be as little as a single paragraph listing possible contraindications (side effects.) Three years later, there can be two or three pages of problems listed based on the harmful side effects - and possible demise - observed in the patients who have been tested in the marketplace with the drug.

This situation clearly violates medicine's Hippocratic Oath and the admonition of "do no harm."

Our current chemical approach to maladies has guided me to believe that the very medication employed potentially aggravates normal bio-frequency pathways which may ultimately be found to be the causative reason for side-effects.

Today, science observes the negative effect of the chemical medication on the biochemistry of the patient, assuming it is the very drug that is causing side effects.[144] Chemistry, which is altered biology, not coming from organic elements breaks the electromagnetic chain that governs your inherent meridian (anatomical wiring system) health.

In my work, continual observation of measurable electromagnetic changes when one is either on or off medications has led me to this conclusion. Drilling down even further, when one is consuming chemically latent (pesticides, fungicides, herbicides, and GMOs) "food" there are detectable, abnormal wavelengths that are measurable with biofeedback technology.

These same individuals can be tested after adopting an uncooked, organic, plant-based diet and, within as little as 18 days, no longer display the same anomalies. These outcomes are consistent with the work of Germany's Popp and America's Hunt from the 20th century.

With the Hunt Meter's approach to measuring energy fields, there is no intrusive harm being inflicted on the person being evaluated. Equally important, the Meter reading will enable a practitioner to begin a correction of the disturbance in the energy field. Once the field is corrected, a person's symptoms can disappear, and healing can occur, unlike with 'modern' medicine and its fixation with the alleviation of symptoms, an obsession that too often results in a return of the disease.

Another persistent mystery about the healing process has been the question of why some people heal successfully and other people fail. Why do spontaneous remissions of disease occur for some people, and these same conditions end up killing other people who could have recovered?

The answer to these and other vexing questions may be found in Dr. Hunt's research and her identification of a synergistic process she calls 'healing transaction.'[145] There are five interconnecting factors that play a role in who will be healed, by what method, and with which healer.

- Energy field of the disease;
- Energy field of the person with that disease;
- Energy field of the healer or physician;
- Energy field of the therapy being used as treatment;
- Combined energy fields of the healer with the type of therapy being used.

Both the patient and the practitioner must co-create the healing field to move and change a patient's disordered energy field. The energy field of the expert combined with that of the treatment being used must be in alignment with the patient for healing results to occur.

In 'conventional' medicine, we have always heard about the effects of a physician's 'bedside manner' on a patient's mental and emotional state. The conventional wisdom has been that a physician can project both conscious and unconscious signals to a patient that help to shape the patient's healing outlook and will to live.[146] Bernie Segal, MD., as well as Patch Adams, MD. both vividly exposed the powerful effect that loving care has on patients. In most medical schools, there is no time spent on pastoral exchange.

Yet there are hundreds of hours spent on prescribing medicine. Today's sick society has exhausted medical faculties globally. Even the most well-intentioned physicians and nurses are not afforded the time to spend with their patients.

Over decades, thousands of times, I have heard hospitals described as cold, impersonal assembly line factories. Humanity is literally at stake and it is time to reevaluate how we perceive and address disease. Dr. Hunt's research takes this understanding to a whole new level.

Because the healer physician has an individual Signature Field, some will be a great help with pain but are energetically unable to regenerate tissue. Their energy field is quite specific to the type of healing they are most effective at. The Aura Meter can help to pair a patient with the most effective practitioner. Those with the most innate ability can actually change, either consciously or intuitively, their own energy field based on the energy field needs of their patient.

Reported 'energy' healings that produce remissions and radical regenerations are low-level transfers of a subtle form of positive radiation that might simply trigger the body's own inherent healing powers.

Most energy practitioners believe that they channel, rather than generate, healing energy.[147] By taking ego out of the healing equation as much as possible, they are more able to summon compassion for their clients. Compassion is a nourishment from which health can grow.

Healing powers of intention

By focusing the attention of the mind toward achieving a healing result, feelings of compassion might be amplified. Such a phenomenon can also be summoned and harnessed during traditional healing rituals and practices. In self-healing practices, intention and focus via breathing allow the flow of energy to resume its healing path. Several laboratory studies demonstrate various aspects of this effect.

In a study conducted at the California Pacific Medical Center, cultured human brain cells showed a sharp increase in growth when treated by the intentions of energy practitioners, compared to a control group.

In a second study, okra and black zucchini squash seeds were placed inside of Petri dish growth chambers at the University of Arizona, with one group given healing intention energy from practitioners to encourage growth, and the control group receiving no attention. Seeds receiving the intentional healing treatments germinated and grew by a rate 20 percent faster and more plentiful than the control group.[148] To test the effects of 'compassionate intention' when it was sent to a 'receiver' by a 'sender,' 22 couples were recruited by a team of scientists from the Institute of Noetic Science, University of Washington School of Medicine, and four other medical institutions. One person in each of the couples was a cancer patient receiving treatment for the disease. Each person was open to the process. These couples were divided into two groups: the first had a person from each couple trained on how to direct compassionate intention toward the patient, while a second group of couples received no training. As the recipient from each couple relaxed in a reclining chair, isolated in a distant steel-walled, electromagnetically shielded room, the sending person repeatedly emitted 10-second bursts of directed intention. Meanwhile, skin conductance and other physiological variables were measured with electrodes in all of the study participants, as they attempted to feel the presence of their partner.

The meter indicated that energy fields heightened when people projected compassionate intentions. Results showed that measurements of the receiver's skin conductance "were the largest and most sustained in the trained group," those who had learned the skill of projecting their compassionate intentions. "Directing intention toward a distant person is correlated with activation of that person's autonomic nervous system," concluded the research team. "Strong motivations to heal and be healed, and training on how to cultivate and direct compassionate intention, may further enhance this effect."[149] Distant healing intention, as the process is called in the medical literature, was taught to the healthy partners in these study couples during a daylong, eight-hour group workshop. "The program included a lecture on the healing potential of compassionate intention, discussion of common resistance to positive expectations about distant healing intention, guided instruction in several meditations and mental focusing practices, and guided exercises in breath-based techniques for enhancing compassion."

After attending this short workshop, healthy partners were encouraged to practice the distant healing meditation daily for three months, before they actually used it on their partner during the experiment. This helped the participants to be effective healers. On the day of the experiment, couples were asked to maintain a "feeling of connectedness" with each other by exchanging personal items, such as watches or rings, and to hold that item during the session.

These feelings of human connectedness have parallels in the realm of physics. Quantum Entanglement holds that elementary particles, once in contact, appear to continue influencing each other after they separate, regardless of the distance. This helps to explain the long-held belief, via observation that "long-term, highly motivated, bonded couples," as the research team wrote, influence each other physiologically, using their minds to project compassionate intention.[150]

Lab Tests of Edd Edwards

Perhaps the most remarkable living channel of bioenergies, as measured in laboratory testing, is Edd Edwards, whom I have worked with at Hippocrates. Edd is a phenomenon who promotes self-healing and who has been studied for his ability to manipulate his bioenergies. He is considered a "Bio-Intrinsic Resonant Energy Specialist" controlling, at will, the human bio-electric field of energy.[151] As a child in northern Georgia, Edd was taught to perceive human bioenergy fields by his grandmother, who was recognized in her community for her ability to assist neighbors with health issues. She counseled Edd on the nature of a personal energy field within his body, and told him he would "have to learn on his own how to develop it."

His Grandmother was right. For thirty years, Edd worked to develop this energy within him, growing increasingly more skillful. However, he found little in the way of outside support. "I spoke with science teachers, community elders, and others. Unfortunately, this search was fruitless" as Edd recounted. Until, upon seeing a CBS television special report in 1994, in which Dr. William Levengood was interviewed about the human energy phenomenon. Edd felt this might be what he possessed. So, he contacted Levengood at the University of Michigan, and eventually became one of this progressive doctor's research subjects.

Since that time, Edd has undergone repeated testing and observation. He has been monitored by a device called a biophoton multiplier that measures the biophoton energetic output coming from his neurological system. He demonstrated an uncanny ability to control this energetic output from his energy field. The more he worked with researchers, the more he was able to learn how to focus and project his bioenergy at will.

Edd calls what he does a projection of "Bio-Intrinsic Resonant Energy," a universal energy where he acts as a conduit. This can be harnessed to activate healing mechanisms within each person. He believes that anyone can learn, with enough practice, how to work with these energies. People who already do Qigong or Tai Chi, ancient practices that most resemble what Edd does, seem to have the easiest time mastering a resonance with these fields of energy.

Starting in 2014, Edd began working in a lab setting with two scientists at the forefront of this bioenergy research --- electrical engineer Ross Dunseath, Ph.D., and neuroscientist Edward Kelly, Ph.D., both at the University of Virginia's Division of Perceptual Studies. In addition, Edd had previously been studied extensively at the Rhine Research Center., Durham, North Carolina. In a December 26, 2015 newsletter, published by the Rhine Center, scientific evaluations of Edd and his performance in the Rhine Bioenergy Lab, were described:

"Edd has been one of the most consistent and effective participants in the studies at the Rhine Bioenergy Lab. In early research, Edd produced results indicating an ability to generate measurable energies at levels much higher than any other participants. While the average energetic output measured in photons of ultraviolet light is between 12-20 photons per second, some gifted participants produced 80 photons, 200 photons, and sometimes even up to 1200 photons per second, while in periods of meditation or while practicing energetic healing."

These results are rare, and statistically significant. Though they are impressive, these results do not compare with Edd's laboratory sessions. Edd has been consistently projecting 2000, 300,000, and sometimes over 1 million photons per second in the lab. In addition, it was clear in the studies that Edd was able to consciously control his energetic output." Though his healing abilities have not been confirmed in the Rhine labs," the Rhine newsletter continued, "he has worked with medical professionals at many different institutions to assist in the comfort and healing of patients. In addition, many people have provided testimonials of the effects they have received from Edd's treatment and of positive health benefits after their sessions with Edd."

Lab studies of Edd by a team of scientists continued at Rhine until 2018.[152] One ongoing area of research involves the specific makeup of the energies he produces, and where those energies originate from within his body.

CHAPTER 10:

Nourish Your Cells, Replenish Your Energy Field

"Food is not just calories, it is information. It talks to your DNA and tells it what to do. The most powerful tool to change your health, environment, and the entire world is your fork." – Mark Hyman, M.D.

"Human nutrition is founded on the Sun's energy rendered through plants...we humans derive energy from the sun through the photosynthesis of plants...our genes teach us that fresh foods taste better and they impart more life energy...to understand energy at the cellular level, we need to know that inside the cells are specific power generating organelles called mitochondria. These energy generators are necessary for the life of practically every kind of cell in our bodies...Mitochondria make the pure chemical energy of life."

This insight into the central role of health at the cellular level comes from a book by Jack Tips, *The Healing Power Within: The Story of Natural Healing and Cellular Energy*. [153] Tips, who holds a doctorate in nutritional science, wrote:

"When there is a lack of cellular energy, there are inevitable problems: the body ages more rapidly, tissues fail, hormones become less effective, arteries become hard, cellular communications get garbled, inflammation becomes chronic, fat gets stored, the brain systems become sluggish, the immune system becomes confused and pathogens create problems. With the human body, low cellular energy always leads to one disease or another...We live and die at the cellular level. Either we have Life energy or the cells perish." Picture your body as a pristine battery filled with maximum energy. This power is provided for us via living, plant-based food, a positive motivational attitude, and rigorous movement and exercise. This triune of affirmative input is required to maintain a high level of frequency, filling that battery to the brim. This is my core work with people who often are enduring catastrophic diseases. When they embrace and apply these simple principles, they have the ability to melt away disorders, open up cluttered biological pathways, and begin to thrive, not just survive.

Cross-section of Mitochondria

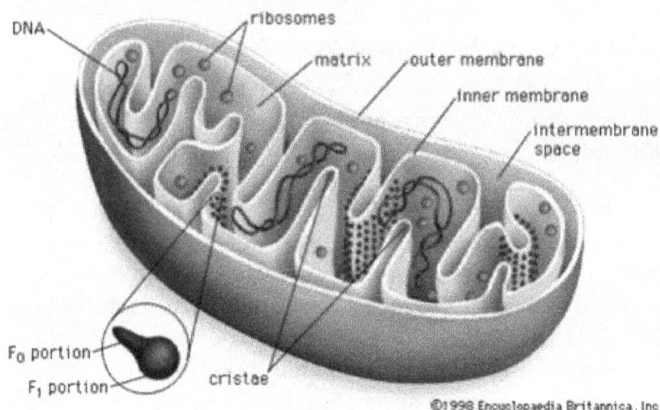

©1998 Encyclopaedia Britannica, Inc.

"The production of energy requires a good diet of whole, natural foods— plant proteins, fats, and carbohydrates that are replete with all their trace minerals and micro nutrients that nature provides. This means that every time you eat whole food—raw vegetables, raw seeds, ripe fresh fruit, raw nuts, etc. you are getting all the compliments of nature[154] and its powerful bio-frequency."

The Tapestry of Life

Magnetites are magnetic particles contained in all cells[155] that directly connect you to all other magnetic fields. Oxygen, water, protein, vitamins, minerals, and essential fatty acids are examples of elements with varied frequencies, and they are attracted to the magnetic energy of the cell. This allows building and life-maintaining processes to engage. This also helps the cell with cleansing the waste from the cell and slowing apoptosis (expected natural cell death).

Unfriendly microbes, like viruses, have an innate ability to use human cells as their hosts. Their manner of functioning is a double-edged sword: viruses strengthen our anatomical resolve by engaging our immune system, while at the same time, we have to battle that virus, making us more vulnerable to that microbe and other disorder.

Disease occurs when the immune system fails. Many researchers and physicians like Dr. Judy Mikovits on the cutting edge of cancer exploration now believe that viruses weaken the integrity of healthy cells enough to be the central cause of cancers.[156] When combined with poor lifestyle habits, a plethora of man-made chemicals that pervade the environment combined with psychological missteps, it is no wonder that cancer is now one of the deadliest diseases we humans encounter.[157]

Our brains are made up of fat, water, and the balance of approximately half neurons and half glial cells.[158] When lacking vital nutrients, the cells falter, creating abnormal psychological and biological concerns. Proper cell function is the basis of a healthy brain.

We are rich with vibrational life in each of the trillions of cells that make up our bodies. This life must be maintained at a high frequency, or we begin to stumble at every level.

Each microorganism, most of which are invisible, contributes to the tapestry of wholeness that makes up our planetary ecosystem. This ecosystem can only flourish when each of these organisms is acknowledged and supported for its contributions.

Inside your cells, there is a limitless network of subcultures. Each subculture has a purposeful role: to charge itself and connect with all other cells. This foundational biology literally creates our entire skeletal structure and various organ systems. We must assure our bodies that we are good caretakers or they will fall into disarray and inevitably disease.

Electrical currents may be key in preventing and remedying maladies. There may well be "electronic switching and transmission systems within and between cells," observed Richard Gerber, M.D., in his book, *Vibrational Medicine.* He bases this observation on findings by Dr. Robert O. Becker, an orthopedic surgeon in New York, who showed how electrical currents within the nervous system foster tissue repair and regeneration.

Our ability to utilize advanced technologies that employ electrical currents will revolutionize the field of healthcare. Dr. Gerber stated, "Perhaps the most revolutionary application of electrotherapy is in stimulating the body's innate capacity for tissue regeneration...The most widespread application of Becker's research, has been in the area of accelerated healing of bone fractures by externally applied electromagnetic fields."[159]

A Role for Quantum Processes

In their book, *Life on the Edge: The Coming Age of Quantum Biology,* Johnjoe McFadden[160] (a molecular geneticist) and Jim Al-Khalili [161] (a theoretical physicist) discussed enzymes as the engines of life (responsible for digestion, respiration, photosynthesis, and metabolism), and how quantum mechanics "plays a key role in the action of at least some if not all enzymes."

The following are excerpts from their book:

1 "It seems that life's catalysts are able to reach down into a deeper level of reality than plain old classical chemistry and make use of some neat quantum trickery...As we have discovered, one of the key activities of enzymes is to move electrons around within substrate molecules, as for example when collagenase pushes and pulls electrons within the peptide molecule. But as well as being pushed around within molecules, electrons can also be transferred from one molecule to another."

2 "Enzymes have made and unmade every single biomolecule inside every living cell that lives or has ever lived. Enzymes are as close as anything to the vital factors of life. So, the discovery that some, and possibly all, enzymes work by promoting the dematerialization of particles from one point in space and their instantaneous materialization in another provides us with a novel insight into the mystery of life. And while there remain many unresolved issues related to enzymes that need to be better understood, such as the role of protein motions, there is no doubt that quantum tunneling (connections) plays a role in the way they work."

3 "Chlorophyll is probably the second most important molecule on our planet after DNA...By comparing photosynthesis in plants with the respiration (burning our food/fuel) that takes place in our own cells, you can see that, under the skin, animals and plants are not so different. The essential distinction lies in where we, and they, get the fundamental building blocks of life. Both need carbon, but plants obtain it from air whereas we get it from organic sources, such as the plants themselves. Both need electrons to build biomolecules; we burn organic molecules to capture their electrons, while plants use light to burn water to capture its electrons. And both need energy; we scavenge it from the high energy electrons that we obtain from our food by running them down respiratory energy hillsides; plants capture the energy of solar photos. Each of these processes involves the motion of fundamental particles that are governed by quantum rules. Life seems to be harnessing quantum processes to help it along."[67]

Your Cells are the Epicenter of Change

Raw, living plant-based foods contain micro-currents of electromagnetic frequency that positively affect red blood and immune system cells to strengthen and protect health. Life starts with light from the electromagnetic spectrum streaming directly from the sun. This light is then transmuted into different levels of frequency, creating unique structures of matter, the most essential being in the plant kingdom.

Nutritional science, as practiced in the mainstream, remains stuck in the dark ages when it comes to connecting our nutrients to sunlight. Plants are matter-based particles of energy from the sun. The human body yearns for the microcurrent frequencies that manifest in the nutrient particles. Higher frequencies increase the body's own electromagnetic field and allow all cells, particularly the immune system, to function at optimal levels.

We are vessels of light particle assimilation and emission. The only materials that pass through the cell phosphorous sheaths are the light particles of vitamins, minerals, nutrients, and unfortunately man-made chemical elements. In other words, phosphorus is a mineral that helps to hold us in physical form by bonding with oxygen in the body[162], which then covers and protects our cells.

When isolated from all other chemical components, phosphorus makes a hissing sound and disappears from this dimension. Phosphorous absorbs light and transmutes those light waves in slow time sequences to different frequencies thus creating the state of phosphorescence, or being biologically, energetically charged.

From 1988 until 2008 here at the Hippocrates Health Institute, we conducted microscopic cell testing on 50,000 participants. Each of these individuals was adhering to a strictly raw, unprocessed, plant-based, and raw plant supplement-consuming diet. With no exception, there were significant increases in biofrequency of individual cells that visibly corrected abnormal functioning to be replaced by optimal performance.

What this indicates is the pinnacle necessity for the repletion of electrical charge. Although proteins, vitamins, minerals, and essential fats are addressing the structural need of cell and tissue development, the frequency governs the core purpose of this biological process. Peptides, phytochemicals, and other elemental factors interact with the network of circuitry that is fed by the consumed electrical charge of food harmonizing with the naturally occurring frequencies developed by the mechanics of the organ systems.

All disease and premature aging are accomplished by having renegade electrons (free radicals) attack healthy and vital cells. When the plasma's charge is less than ideal, the individual cells are easily killed, creating a cascade of cellular demise.

Quantum medicine must apply the foundational principle that diseases can be prevented and even reversed by enhancing the internal and external shields around our cells. Now in our seventh decade of conducting daily clinical observation on people in the throes of serious illness, we have established a definitive pattern exposing the necessity of electron vitality.

The UCLA experiments conducted by Professor Valerie Hunt documented a dull radiation that flows from the body of someone eating junk food. All such foods are lifeless in vibration, dead, quiet, and inert, being unable to reproduce life. These so-called 'foods' do not feed the human energy field. The vibrations are low in frequency and small in amplitude, providing only calories and empty, unneeded chemistry.

Without life-giving electromagnetic energies from consuming living foods, a human's energies remain dull and small. Measurements taken in Dr. Hunt's laboratory also showed layers of expansively multiplying vibrational energy extending from the body when a person consumes plant-based raw food.

These foods nourish the electromagnetic field. Vegetables, sprouted grains, beans, nuts, seeds, and fruit are vibrant living substances that enhance the human energy field. This should be the foremost reason we call these 'healing' foods.

Although the natural state of human food consumption is fresh living and plant-based, most of us have been tainted by lifelong use of processed, chemicalized, genetically modified, and often synthetic food.

To further complicate our relationship with nutrition, are the willing and unscrupulous industries that intentionally infuse these processed products with "hyper palatability"[163] (where the industry adds synthetic opiate substances in to addict the consumer).

Today people's fear-driven consumption is accelerated by the intentional addiction brought forth by the manipulation of these products. Former U.S. FDA head Dr. David Kessler pointed out in his book, *The End of Overeating*, that well over half of the FDA's budget comes from the pharmaceutical and food industries. This is a perfect example of the fox running the henhouse. Kessler also found overwhelming evidence that food scientists hired by corrupt food manufacturers were commissioned to find ways to make processed foods more seductive and addictive. Chemical flavorings are an essential weapon for toxic addiction in the arsenal of the food industry. Kessler asked chef Wolfgang Puck why he thought consumers were overeating and he replied, "Sugar, fat, and salt. People can't get enough."[164] Now we can add intentionally placed addictive chemistry.

Digestion ultimately occurs in the cell. So, it's imperative that we consume only pure and life-filled sustenance. Nourishment that resonates with the total of all life energies also affords you the potential to let go of your old preconceived notions and accept the omnipresent consciousness that abounds. Lacking fulfillment, passion, and focus, people have relegated themselves to the perpetual over-consumption of toxic non-foods for their narcotic effects.

Influential plant-based eaters include Plato, Leonardo DaVinci, Isaac Newton, Benjamin Franklin, women's rights champion Susan B. Anthony, Mahatma Gandhi[165], Henry Ford[166], and the novelist Alice Walker.

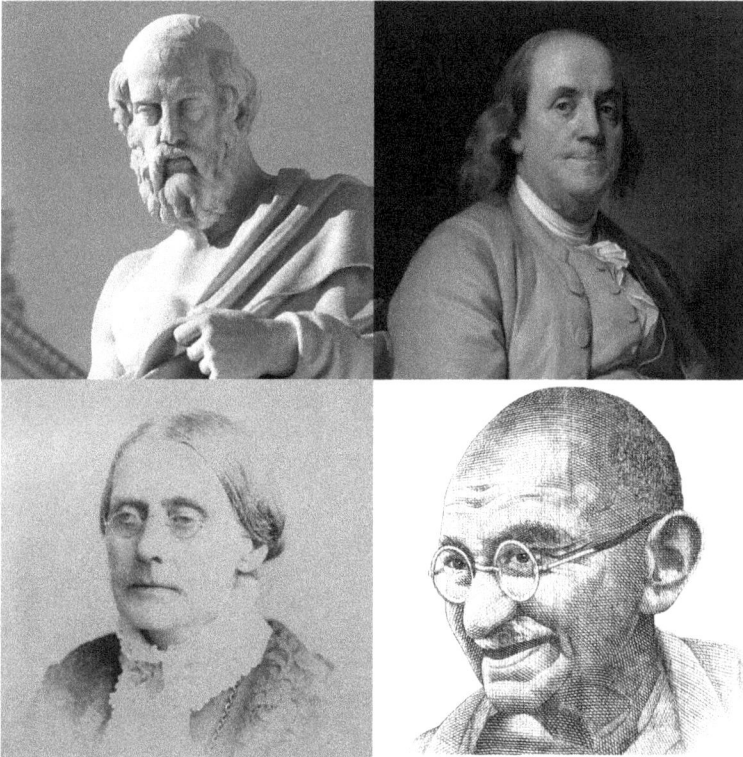

(Top left to bottom right: Plato, Benjamin Franklin, Susan B. Anthony, Mahatma Gandhi).

Although nutrition is paramount in fueling the body. Productive movement and exercise ignite a secondary level of energy that is essential to achieve abundant health. Exercise, walking and physical work create an energy field dynamic in the human body which is vitalizing. When exercise is done outdoors, the fields of growing plants, the wind, and the fresh air, further increase the electromagnetic enhancement of your life force.

Our study observation has been clear in findings and conclusions. Those who partake in the consumption of plant-based food and adopt a more physically active lifestyle open their hearts and minds, dramatically increasing their chances of healing.

Certain nutrients, when amplified by positive thoughts and actions, can help to regenerate the immune system. The pinnacle of the numerous foods we employ in our Hippocrates Institute's lifestyle program is wheatgrass juice, which in great part is chlorophyll, enhancing the ability of red blood cells to carry oxygen. Dozens of lab studies reported in prestigious medical journals show wheatgrass to be effective in preventing and healing disease.

In 1983, Dr. Valerie Hunt used her meter, which was initially developed with her colleagues at the NASA space program to monitor the most subtle energy and frequencies that had ever been evaluated. She used it to conduct research on the electron activity of various edible plants. Determining that the only valid foods with measurable resonant frequency were botanical and not animal sources. Here is the electrical conductivity valuation Dr. Hunt found for each nutrient, in her select top ten plant food categories.

1. Wheatgrass, Sunflower Sprouts, Pea Shoots, Edible Weeds–2500 Hz.

2. Kale, mustard greens, Bok Choy, Chicory–1500 Hz.

3. Mango, Papaya, Lychee Nuts, Mamay, Starfruit—1250 Hz.

4. Kiwi, Oranges, Grapefruit, Tangerines—1100 Hz.

5. Green and Red Leaf Lettuce, Cabbage, Brussel Sprouts, Endive—1050 Hz.

6. Sauerkraut, Kimchi, fermented vegetables (fermented for at least 3 days)—1000 Hz.

7. Sprouted seeds (2 days), Sunflower, Sesame—975 Hz.

8. Sprouted nuts, Almond, Hazel, Pinola—880 Hz.

9. Root vegetables, Turnips, Rutabaga, Jicama, Radish—650 Hz.

10. Vegetables or fruit blended (90 seconds or more) —50 Hz.

(Note to Readers: Fruit consumption should be avoided during any attempt to conquer disease since the high sugar content outweighs the frequency benefit.)

Meta analyses of 17 studies conducted over a 50-year period, in 8 countries, brought to light that a healthy human cell contains 75 Hz. All of the above-mentioned foods, consumed in their fresh and uncooked state and taking into account the energy lost in the digestion and elimination process, render frequencies to assist in cell maintenance.

"Electromagnetic fields exist within each cell, tissue, and organ, and within and around the body as a whole," observed Daniel J. Benor, M.D., in his book, *Consciousness Bioenergy and Healing*. "These are viewed by conventional medicine as the result of electrochemical properties and activities of the cells and tissues. Complementary Medicine therapists suggest that the bioelectrical fields may have a regulating function upon and within the body." [167] Hunt found that each cell has electron activity that connects to all other cells, creating a web, or meridian, which systematically controls anatomical and psychological functions. We believe this web, in turn, connects us to all other life.

Food Energy Verified

One afternoon, I received a call from Dr. Rick Ricketts[168], a renowned orthodontist, who was associated with the University of California. Excitedly, he suggested that we do energy photography on the living foods that we not only consume, but advocate for. At the time, the University had in residence a professor from Russia, who was an expert energy photographer. Soon thereafter, she presented to us a series of enlightening photos of wheatgrass and sunflower sprouts. The accompanying scientific evaluation was stunning. By calculating the extent of energy within the cells of the plants, when spilling over into the surrounding environment it allowed her to precisely measure the flow of frequency. These images showed energy bursting from fresh growing plants; emanating outward two feet in every direction.

In my book, *Living Food for Optimum Health*[169], I published one of these photographs, which verifies that uncooked fresh living foods contain and maintain nearly all of their nutrients and medicines called phytochemicals. Other research, like that of Dr. David Williams[170] at the Linus Pauling Institute, has made similar findings. But more so, fresh living foods maintain energy captured on the leaves of plants pouring from the sun and manifesting through the photosynthesis process.

Fifty years ago, Dr. Valerie Hunt motion-photographed a young student consuming a standard Western diet, showing the effect it had on his body's bio-frequency field. The same student was then placed on raw living food, and as you see in the pictures below, reversed the energy contraction to an expansion, exuding frequency.

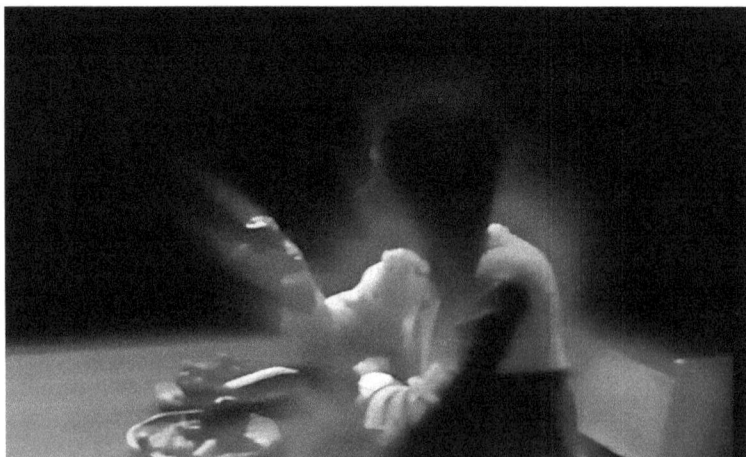

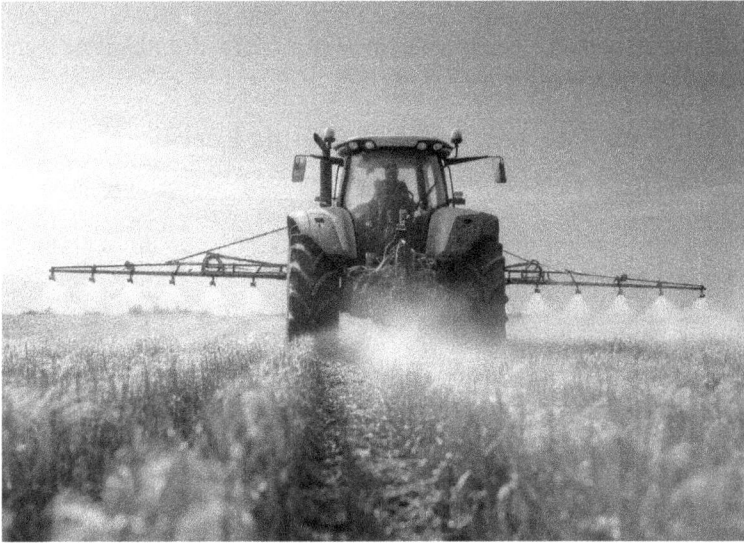

A Russian Physicist Expands the Science

Dr. Konstantin Korotkov[171] is a respected physics professor and researcher in St. Petersburg, Russia. Upon recently contacting him, I suggested that we study the effect that commercial pesticide-riddled food crops have on the energy within the plant. On the opposite end of the spectrum, we wanted to see if there was a difference when food was grown organically. Dr. Korotkov wisely chose a common vegetable, a carrot, to study.

Electrophotonic imaging (EPI)[172], a technique that Dr Korotkov has also used in other studies[173], was utilized in this research. Two samples were taken from carrots, one being free of chemicals, the other a standard commercial variety. Each sample's diameter was 15 mm, thickness. The study was conducted immediately after harvesting. Samples were dried for approximately one hour in a controlled condition, without altering their enzymatic activity. For every sample, 20 tests were conducted and the results were averaged.

There was a statistical significance in the intensity of light emitting from the varying samples. There is no doubt that one of the central causes of many diseases, including tumor and cancer growth, is partly due to the dynamic and dramatic reduction in the bio-frequency field of what we choose to consume. In fact, the conventional scientific community is fast approaching the conclusions we have historically come to at Hippocrates.

The most important antidote for premature aging and disease is natural, by which I mean the naturally occurring bio resonance harvested from organic living edible plants.

Water Conducts and Amplifies Subtle Energies

In a series of experiments, Professor Bernard Grad[175], of Canada's McGill University, tested the effects on barley seeds when they were grown in water 'treated' by humans using only laying-on-of-hands[176]. After soaking barley seeds in salt water, which retards growth, Grad has his test subjects use their hands to 'treat' some of the seeds while other seeds remained untreated. All seeds were then placed in an incubator to study germination and growth. It was found that seeds exposed to energy-treated water sprouted 30 percent more often than those in the saline group.

Next, the seeds from both the treated and untreated groups were potted and growth was monitored. 'Treated' seeds showed significantly greater growth and chlorophyll content after several weeks of observation. Grad replicated these findings numerous times. In a separate experiment, Grad had severely depressed psychiatric patients 'treat' the water used to grow barley seeds and discovered such contact "suppressed the growth rate of seedlings."

Can persons with a 'green thumb,' who seem much more able than others to facilitate plant growth and health, also duplicate what healers did to the barley seeds? Apparently, the answer is yes, because sealed bottles of water treated by 'green thumb' individuals also caused an increased growth rate in the tested plants.

By carrying out chemical analyses of treated versus non-treated water, Grad detected numerous anomalies. Treated water showed a shift in the atomic bond angle of water molecules; decreased hydrogen bonding occurred between water molecules; and a big decrease could be found in the surface tension of treated water. Some of these effects also occurred when water was exposed to magnets, perhaps indicating that human contact with water exerts a magnetic transformation beneficial to plant growth and health.

To further test Grad's findings, a research chemist in Atlanta, Dr. Robert Miller, verified that human energy 'treated' water does disrupt the observed hydrogen bonding in water. Not only that, he discovered striking similarities between these hydrogen effects in both energy treatment and contact with magnetic fields. Water that had been exposed to magnetic fields also showed significant reductions in surface tension, which was similar to what had been observed with healers.

Taking his research a step further, Miller experimentally analyzed the effect of this treated water on the rate of rye seedling germination. He took ordinary tap water and used some as a control, with no treatment, and other water was either exposed to a magnetic field or to human hand treatment and each type of water was applied to groups of 25 rye grass seeds.

After four days of observation, Miller found that "seeds which had been watered with regular tap water had an eight- percent germination rate, whereas seeds watered with human energy-treated water showed a 36 percent germination rate—or a fourfold increase in the number of new sprouts."

"The results of Dr. Miller's and Dr. Grad's studies provided new experimental evidence for the magnetic nature of the energies of healers," observed Richard Gerber, M.D., author of *Vibrational Medicine*. "One theory which seemed plausible was that healers accomplished their acceleration of the normal growth and healing processes of living organisms by speeding up the activities of the cellular enzymes which normally carried out these functions."[177] Additional support for the idea that both healer's hands and strong magnetic fields can accelerate enzyme kinetics came from research carried out by Dr. Justa Smith[178], a biochemist at Rosary Hill College in New York. Using the digestive enzyme trypsin, she found that healers were able to "increase the enzyme reaction rate over time" and that, "the longer the healer held the test tube of enzymes, the more rapid the reaction rate. Similar effects on enzymes had been noted with high-intensity magnetic fields…The type of change in enzyme activity noted after exposure to healers was always in the direction of greater health of the cells and thus the organism." [179] That point was underscored by an experiment in which Dr. Smith used ultraviolet light to damage samples of trypsin enzymes by disrupting their protein structures. A person treated the damaged enzymes with hand contact and Smith found "that the damaged enzymes recovered enzymatic activity and that their activity continued to rise linearly over time with continued exposure to the healing energies." In essence, the person had 'healed' the damaged enzymes.

All of these study findings taken together underscore the subtle energetic properties of water and what grows from water when treated by humans, especially those who have set an intention to channel 'healing energies' through their hands, which in turn transfers these energies into plants to alter their physiology and facilitate growth and health. "It would appear that water can be 'charged' with and then 'store' various types of subtle energies," wrote Dr. Richard Gerber. "Subtle energy of both a beneficial and detrimental nature can be stored, as evidenced by Grad's studies utilizing healers and depressed patients."[180]

"These experiments on the subtle energetic properties of water have relevance in examining the known principles of drug therapy vs. the unknown mechanisms of homeopathy," wrote Dr. Gerber. "When researchers describe the pharmacokinetic theory, it is important to give patients a high enough drug dosage to obtain therapeutic blood levels. Most drugs cause what are known as dose-dependent effects. The higher the amount of drug given, the more potent the physiological effects."

"Conversely, in homeopathy, the more dilute the drug dosage the more powerful its effects. Drug solutions used to make homeopathic remedies are so dilute they are unlikely to contain even single molecules of the original substance, yet they appear to have powerful healing effects." What homeopathy may be doing is "matching the frequency of the plant extract with the frequency of the illness."

"Homeopathic remedies represent an alternative evolutionary pathway in the application of medicinal plant therapies. Where pharmacologists chose to isolate single, active molecular agents from herbs, homeopaths worked with the vibrational essence of the whole plant substance. The homeopathic preparation process liberates from the plants the subtle energetic qualities to charge water, from which they are then transferred to tinctures for individualized dosage."

Still another vibrational approach identified by Dr. Gerber, "which represents a radical offshoot from herbal medicine, is based on the administration of flower essences. As with homeopathic remedies, the preparation of these essences is dependent upon the subtle energetic storage properties of water. Bach Flower essences also utilize the subtle properties of sunlight to imprint upon the medium of water the vibrational qualities of the flowers." [87]

CHAPTER 11:

Thoughts Channel Healing Energy

"If someone wishes for good health, one must first ask oneself if he is ready to do away with the reasons for his illness. Only then is it possible to help him." - Hippocrates 370 BC

Negative thoughts and fear will strip your power, making you vulnerable to seduction by toxic cultural forces. Positive thoughts, by contrast, transcend matter and provide endless energy to overcome unhealthy influences. Self-awareness and focus have the ability to foster optimal health.

"Mind resides on some non-physical plane(s), but expresses itself via transformations of energy or information through the brain," observed Daniel J. Benor, M.D., in Consciousness Bioenergy and Healing.[186] "The brain contains an estimated 10 to 14 billion nerve cells, with a constant interplay of electrochemical messages between its countless interconnections. It is possible that the brain may readily be influenced by outside energies that can modulate some of this ongoing intercellular activity. A minimum of energy input might be required to influence any of the multitudes of brain cells that are frequently standing on the threshold of emitting impulses. Thus the brain would act like a radio or TV receiver."

Currently, exploration in consciousness is how the quantum effect manifests. Nobel laureate Sir Roger Penrose and his colleague Dr. Stuart Hameroff created what is now known as Orch OR[187], which measures gravitational instabilities in the fundamental structure of space-time collapse. Quantum Wave functions in tiny structures called Microtubules. These minute yet essential functionaries are found inside of neurons. Several groups of advanced quantum researchers dotting the globe are finding that this may just be the way that we can eventually duplicate consciousness.

In the year 2023, Aarat Kalra and Gregory Scholes, physical chemist / Princeton University, led a study[188] on how energy absorbs in the form of light. Remarkably this propagates within microtubules.

Another team led by Na Li at Huazhong University of Science and Technology in Wuhan, China, did mouse studies using four different isotopes of Xenon gas[189]. The isotopes containing an odd number of neutrons in their nucleus gave them a quantum property called "Spin." When using the anesthetics effect there was a 20 % differential with the quantum effect, furthering Penrose's and Hameroff's work.

Biophysicist Dr. Luca Turin at the University of Buckingham, U.K., and Dr. Kenneth Kosik at the University of California at Santa Barbara, point out that brain organoids[190] comprised of several million cells in a ball about the size of a lentil can be grown in a laboratory mimicking what happens during the natural growth of embryos.

Brain organoids are much easier to probe when using a recording system, they show that neurons wire themselves up spontaneously. Alysson Muotori[191], University of California San Diego states "As far as we can tell they make connections they would naturally do in the brain."

We are slowly edging closer to dissecting and realizing what consciousness is. Our brain's so-called biological computer, often called a "radical pair," is considered the poster child of Quantum biology.

When studying birds and their eyes and how they navigate globally, the thinking is that the birds' sensitivity to the way the microtubules inside the neurons interrelate to electrons is what allows the creature to know if they are flying north or south. Previously, we thought it was gravity's ion cord that guided them north, south, east, or west. Now, it appears it is internal consciousness.

Christoph Simon, a physicist at the University of Calgary, Canada, states that after all of this international data is reviewed and analyzed the Orch Or process is far more plausible. We will soon understand the inner workings of internal consciousness and how it connects with universal awareness.

When this is achieved it will enable science to guide people into the world that surrounds us in a larger, brighter and more comprehensive way. Today every human residing on earth has limited vision. It is very rare that one can accelerate to the level where they change from matter to frequency connecting them to the greater electromagnetic current that is the multiple and endless universes. Imagine a time when we eradicate our fear that limits our abilities and become as whole happy and functional as we are meant to be.

Our energy fields are organized by our emotions, particularly our 'soul' emotions from the past with their accompanying bio-energy fields. Sometimes these leftover soul emotions are so painful that the person cannot transact with a practitioner in a healing process. Unresolved emotions causing turmoil will continue to affect the field. This unifying network connects you to the timeless, endless multi-universe, at all times in a continuum.

Movement, music, and inner imagery techniques are all useful in the healing process. Depending on the patient's pattern of anti-coherent frequencies, one type of healing requires slow, flowing motions, while another may need rapid or sporadic motions. When you release forced thoughts and allow your heart frequency to connect to sound, light, or movement, you tune into the inherent library of wisdom that sparks healing.

The Number One Mystery

Every few years the British science magazine *New Scientist*[192] compiles a list of the most intriguing mysteries of life and the universe. With regularity such puzzling phenomena as 'dark matter,' cold fusion, and ultra-energetic cosmic rays show up alongside ten other "situations that do not make scientific sense," ranked by the magazine from one through thirteen according to how much of a dilemma they pose for mainstream scientists and their prevailing theories of how everything works.

Each time this survey has been compiled in the 21st century, the number one spot has been occupied by a seemingly mundane phenomenon that any one of us can experience – the placebo effect – which affronts the rational sensibilities of scientists with the question of why a whole lot of "nothing" can still be a very powerful force.

As it is conventionally defined, a placebo is any unproven medical treatment without known pharmacological action to treat a patient's disease or other medical condition[193]. It can be a sugar pill, a saline solution injection, or an elaborate ritual and/or ruse designed to look like real surgery.

It is a deception, according to the 'mainstream' medicine point of view, whose only real usefulness comes in double-blind clinical studies testing the effectiveness of new pharmaceutical drugs. Because mainstream medical science has no workable theory to explain placebo on the body, its positive impact on patients is often ignored or trivialized as random error or 'noise,' as if it were nothing more than a pseudo-science dependent on superstitious beliefs.

Medical professionals have probably conducted more research on the placebo effect than on all the world's pharmaceutical drugs combined, yet investigators are no closer to a concurrent scientific explanation of why the phenomenon works so well in so many people.

Why do 60 percent of all gastric ulcer patients, for instance, claim cures after taking placebo tablets made of sugar?[194][195] How can a simple pill made from carbohydrates relieve the symptoms of a pounding headache? What explains the large numbers of people with degenerative knee conditions who were given fake arthroscopic surgeries and who afterward began to walk normally again[196] without any pain? What explains why placebos can even have side effects like pharmaceutical drugs?

A case in point comes from a study in a 1983 issue of the *World Journal of Surgery* that described how one-third of all people in a placebo control group who thought they were getting a new chemotherapy drug, spontaneously lost all of their hair because they believed chemotherapy was supposed to result in hair loss.[197]

Does Belief Create its Own Reality?

An innovative cancer researcher in Israel, Dr. Gershom Zajicek[198], who regularly utilizes the placebo principle as part of his 'wisdom of the body' prescriptions for treating cancer and inducing remissions, describes the history of medical treatments as a history of the placebo effect, which he further defines as the "successful manipulation of unexplained processes." Rather than denigrate placebos as irrational and unscientific, as most of his colleagues have done, he has become a pioneer in stressing the importance of using placebo treatments for advanced diseases, not only to reduce anxiety and pain, but to jumpstart the body's own natural disease-fighting and self-healing mechanisms. "The placebo effect is the healing force of nature," emphasizes Dr. Zajicek. "It triggers (the body's) natural response."[199]

Why Does the Placebo Effect Make Medical Science Nervous?

Doctors and scientists tend to be cerebrally gifted and are adherents to the systems they study. This education does not leave room for artistic pursuit but is unforgiving in its rigidity and step-by-step approach. When these professionals are faced with "unprovable" situations that have affirmative outcomes, they feel at a loss and tend to disregard the success since they have no control over its process.

Placebo remains a convenient catch-all term, sometimes treated like a medical wastebasket, into which physicians and scientists dismiss anything they cannot readily explain, especially healings that do not fit the Western allopathic model of how healing is supposed to work.

Because placebos involve self-deceit and even ignorance, they are effective due to beliefs, a process that also makes physicians nervous due to the ethical questions that arise about when to inform a patient that a placebo is being used for their own benefit. A 2004 *British Medical Journal* study conducted in Israel found that 62 percent of all physicians surveyed in that country regularly prescribe placebos (including verbal and/or non-medicinal substitute treatments) to their unknowing patients.[200] Another aspect to ponder is about whether the patients are being charged pharmaceutical drug rates for inexpensive sugar and salt pills. Needless to say, whatever the cost, if the results are positive, maybe it is appropriate to ponder ethical consideration.

Fingerprints of the Placebo Effect

Trust, inspired by a physician may make the practitioner the most powerful placebo of all, unfortunately this can result in either affirmative or negative outcomes. These results were reported in the 1987 study in the *British Medical Journal*. When a physician provides patients with a diagnosis and assures them recovery will occur in a few days, 64 percent do recover, in comparison to only a 39 percent recovery rate if the physician claims not to know the cause of the illness or how long it will persist.[201]

Harvard University cardiologist Dr. Herbert Benson[202] has renamed the placebo effect 'remembered wellness'[203] to give it a more acknowledged and prominent role in the healing process of mainstream medicine.

The various amplifying effects of attitudes and behaviors build upon the placebo to produce healing synergies. When a physician's confidence generates a placebo response in the patient, for example, it can amplify the other healing forces of imagination and the power of suggestion.

Keep in mind that this is all due to the ability of a person to tap into the energetic source of all life. No chemistry or procedure is directly used, only acceptance of an energetic shift.

Why has the magnitude of the placebo effect increased over the past few decades? A pioneering scientist provides an answer based on human expectations and intentions interacting with an information entanglement process straight out of quantum physics.

Drug Effectiveness May Be Largely Due
To The Placebo Effect

At least 40 percent or more of any drug's effectiveness is due to the placebo effect, researchers calculate, and that percentage has been growing over the past decade. "The vast majority of drugs – more than 90 percent – only work in 30 to 50 percent of people," revealed Dr. Allen Roses[204], former Worldwide Vice President for the pharmaceutical giant, GlaxoSmithKline, as reported by The Independent in 2003.[205]

If the placebo effect is subtracted from Roses' estimate, does this mean that the pharmaceutical industry is mostly marketing an illusion of effectiveness? With antidepressant drugs, for instance, one medical journal surveyed more than 50 studies on their effectiveness and estimated that up to 75 percent of their reported positive effects are directly due to the placebo effect.[206]

Subliminal messaging from media advertising consistently touts messages about how the medicines they sell will make your disorder disappear and enhance the joy in your life. All of this visual and auditory stimulation intensifies the placebo effect by raising people's expectations and heightening their initial results when the drug is consumed.

If a placebo is a form of trickery, how can we 'trick' ourselves in order to self-administer a placebo treatment and take advantage of its healing properties?

We each have within us our own internal pharmacy. With enough belief, faith, and training, we can learn to release these healing agents in us to relieve ailments and bolster our immunity to illness and disease.

A Theory That Links the Placebo and the Quantum Field

My hypothesis is founded upon research by Dr. David Felten, a neuroscientist, and his team. They discovered that nerve fibers extend into every organ where immune cells are present. This anatomically exposes how thoughts can activate energetic and chemical cascades resulting in biochemical, psychological, and ultimately healing processes. [207]

Others who search for the answer to how mind over matter works have a wide variety of intriguing theories. One gentleman who has currently popularized the power of thought is Dr. Joe Dispenza. In his 2014 book, *You Are the Placebo: Making Your Mind Matter*[208], Dispenza made a compelling case that the placebo effect, particularly as it relates to healing the human body, relies upon an interaction between the quantum mind and quantum fields.

Here at the Institute, we are globally known for the countless number of people that have come to learn and adopt our program and have gone on to reverse their disease. Over decades we have refined our knowledge and understanding of how attitudinal change is often the most important ingredient in conquering disorder. Our faculty includes precision psychotherapists and PhD. psychologists who are acutely interested in shifting one's worries to their strengths.

Every guest who moves through our Life Transformation Program receives individual and group therapy sessions. By merely expressing their pain and unresolved issues, their immune systems immediately engage interferons, interleukins, and activate the fighter cells (Natural Killer cells). Once the positive process begins, the objective is to replace grief with forgiveness, in and of itself this landmark shift sparks the internal orchestrated chemistry required to heal.

The Comprehensive Cancer Wellness[209] program led by Dr. Janet Hranicky, specifically and explicitly addresses pre-cancer traumas, revealing the emotional shift that potentially activated the mutation of cells. Once this desperate circumstance has been acknowledged the important work of retracing and washing away negative patterns can begin. Beyond the human-to-human discussion, we utilize technology like NuCalm, which electronically enables these ill, traumatized individuals to move into a deep state of brain release. The Beta and Alpha states that are layers in what was once called the subconscious harbor the switches that release immune cell activation. When professionally guided, the individual can literally move those fighter cells into the very area where their disease resides.

Although we are seen as ground-breaking pioneers in the burgeoning field of psychoneuroimmunology, we are positive that the future model of disease reversal will intricately involve mind alteration via talk and technology.

Here are some excerpts: "While we may not know exactly how many medical healings are due to the placebo effect (modern-day research shows it can range anywhere from 10 to 100 percent), the overall number is certainly extremely significant. Given that, we have to ask ourselves, *what percentage of diseases and illnesses are due to the effects of negative thoughts in the nocebo?* Considering that the latest research in psychology estimates that about 70 percent of our thoughts are negative and redundant, the number of unconsciously created nocebo-like illnesses might be impressive indeed—certainly much higher than we realize."

"Although it may seem incredible that your mind could actually be that powerful, the research of the past several decades clearly points to a few empowering truths: What you think is what you experience, and when it comes to your health, that's made possible by the amazing pharmacopeia that you have within your body that automatically and exquisitely aligns with your thoughts. This miraculous dispensary activates naturally occurring healing molecules that already exist within."

To activate the placebo response, we must create a new belief, such as the belief *that I will heal myself from this disease.* In Dispenza's words, "The amplitude or energy of that choice must be high enough that it's greater than the hardwired programs and emotional conditioning in the body." Your will to heal must be stronger than the force of your disorder.

"When you change your energy, you change your state of being," writes Dispenza. "Once you fix your attention or your awareness or your mind on possibility, you place your energy there as well. As a result, you're affecting matter with your attention or observation. The placebo effect is not fantasy then; its quantum reality."

Our physical universe "shares a field information (the quantum field) that unifies matter and energy…When you change your energy to alter a belief or perception about yourself or your life, you're actually increasing the frequency of the atoms and molecules of your physical body so that you're amplifying your energy field…so according to the quantum model of reality, we could say that all disease is a lowering of frequency."

"When you change your energy because you made a decision with firm intention, you increase the frequency of your atomic structure and create a more intentional, coherent electromagnetic signature. You're now affecting the physical matter in your body."

As director of Hippocrates Wellness, I have created an energy medicine department where we provide advanced techniques to release obstructive thoughts that precipitate physical and emotional disorders. Each and every person who attends any of our programs receives personal as well as group sessions and energy treatments in the quest for advanced mind solutions. In the case of cancer, we have initiated the Comprehensive Cancer Wellness Protocol Program that heavily relies on the latest science of mind over matter disease reversal. The program's medical director guides this four-week offering. She was a key member of Dr.

Simonton's team and traveled the globe, only working with Stage 4 cancer patients. Calling their technique 'Visualization', they were able to help thousands alter their grim expected outcomes and, in many cases, help the patients reverse their disorder.

Prayer May Affect Species Other Than Just Humans

Healing prayer studies using human subjects have produced mixed results with a dozen or more showing the beneficial impacts of prayer on health, and several other studies showing no effect, which might be explained based on differences in human beliefs, attitudes, and other psychological factors that are difficult to control under experimental conditions.

A study of distant prayer's effects on wound healing in non-human primates, published in the December 2006 peer-reviewed issue of *Alternative Therapies* journal, avoided these issues surrounding the unpredictability of human variables. A science research team at Jackson State University, under a grant from the National Institute of Mental Health, divided 22 bush babies –primates similar to monkeys—into two groups, one was prayed for daily over four weeks by experienced distance healers, while the control group received no prayer attention at all. It was a well-designed, double-blind, randomized study the likes of which had never been conducted before.

During captivity, bush babies tend to over-groom themselves from boredom and stress, causing wounds of various sizes and severity. It is akin to obsessive-compulsive disorder in humans but much more physically self-destructive. After four weeks, the researchers found that the prayer animals had markedly improved wound healing in comparison to the control group. This was calculated by wound size, severity, a reduction in wound grooming time, and a greater increase in red blood cells and hemoglobin. Researchers believe this indicates that the prayer recipients experienced an enhanced oxygen delivery, which accounted for the accelerated wound healing.

"These findings indicate that the phenomenon of prayer appears to be effective in species other than humans," concluded the researchers.[210] Some obvious questions emerge from this research that I will attempt to answer in this book. How can we account for this occurrence? What sort of invisible mechanism is at work?

Traditionally, ancient cultures developed prayer to encourage inspirational, positive thought. Positive thinking has been clinically shown to be a pain reliever. In 2005, in the *Proceedings of the National Academy of Sciences*, a study was published showing how positive thinking can be more powerful than a shot of morphine. Ten volunteers in the study reported they experienced less pain when they expected lower levels of pain, with pain intensity reduced by 28 percent, similar to a dose of the potent painkiller morphine. "Pain needs to be treated with more than just pills," said study co-author Dr. Robert Coghill of Wake Forest University. "The brain can powerfully shape pain and we need to exploit its power."

Certain mental and emotional states have been identified that can help to either combat cancer or even cause its growth. For instance, Professor David Spiegel at Stanford University Medical School did an experiment with 86 women enduring breast cancer in which one group used self-hypnosis to induce a positive state of mind, and the other group did not. Those who received the hypnosis training lived twice as long as the untrained group.

Anomalous Human Energy Effects

Some human beings are naturally so highly charged with energy that they apparently influence the operations of streetlights and other electrical equipment. While these occurrences are mostly anecdotal, and little scientific study or mainstream science attention has been paid to them, so many people have testified to the phenomenon that a book was published chronicling it called *SLIders: The Enigma of Streetlight Interference,* by Hilary Evans[211], under the auspices of the Association for the Scientific Study of Anomalous Phenomena.

Using a database of nearly 200 persons who reported their experiences and filled out questionnaires, Evans reported:

- Both males and females seem to experience it equally;
- The effect is spontaneous and apparently uncontrollable;
- Usually, the effect on electrical equipment occurs within a radius of 30 feet or less from the subject;
- Most often, the person is experiencing strong emotions when the effect happens.

Some reader comments about the book and their experiences with the phenomenon were posted on Amazon.com, and here they are to give you an idea of how widespread these bizarre effects may be. Although there are Sliders worldwide, there are wide variances in the effect they have on electrically charged equipment. Each of these people are obviously wired with an electromagnetic frequency well beyond that of the average person. One of the many stories that impressed me was epitomized in L.Bonner's description.

February 25, 2011

By <u>L. Bonner</u>

I've been waiting for this book for years! I went for many years not putting things together, then more years not realizing there were others like me. One doesn't typically think to ask others if they make watches stop, short out appliances, and erase data from floppy disks by holding them in their hand while in the presence of someone very unbalanced and scary. And others just flat out don't believe you, or tell you what you're claiming is impossible.

I went through a period of extreme stress after my daughter passed away, I became bankrupt, and everything was in a downhill slide for several years. At one point, every time I flipped a switch, I'd fry some device. We had to replace light bulbs on a regular basis. I even came to a point of almost losing a job because I kept fouling up equipment and making track lights explode when I came into my office (they were on a high vaulted ceiling, requiring someone to bring in a tall ladder each time). My most dramatic occurrence happened one morning when I'd had an argument with my husband just before leaving for work. I was fuming. Got into my car and turned the key in the ignition, and all four of my automatic windows started going up and down, at different rates. I kept punching madly at the control buttons on the driver's side door, but they wouldn't stop until I got out of the car. I finally found an online forum one day, with dozens of accounts by other SLIders. What a day of confirmation, relief, and vindication that was! [219]

As discussed, people possessing this unique ability, more often than not, do not share it because, in many instances, when they are discovered by others, they find themselves scrutinized and shunned. This is a perfect example of how we are preventing advancements in our scientific knowledge concerning quantum realms that quite possibly could lead us in a brand-new direction. Luckily, some continue to explore the phenomenon.

During an episode[212] of William Shatner's television series, *Weird or What?* the streetlight phenomenon was featured, and an electrical engineer, Bill Beaty, was interviewed, speculating that some people may be physiologically comparable to walking electric generators. When we inhale, we breathe in electrons from the surrounding air. Something involved with that process may explain why certain people carry around a much more potent electrical charge with the power to short-circuit electrical equipment.

In his book, Evans examined all of the possible explanations for the phenomenon and concluded that persons generating this effect influence "the voltage of the current running through lights and other electrical equipment and it is more likely that it does so by causing a surge... to perform this feat, these highly charged people would have to be an electrodynamic force, somehow generated within or through the human biological system and which transfers into the neighboring environment, where it will act on any appliance which happens to be vulnerable."

Hardcore skeptics insist the phenomenon is nothing more than coincidence (some street lights turn on and off more frequently at the end of their life cycle) combined with wishful thinking on the part of the subject. There may be some truth in that explanation in some cases, but many people who experience the phenomenon say it extends to electrical devices other than street lights. Lamps, cell phones, televisions, and other appliances flick on and off without being touched; volume levels on computers, radios, etc., go up and down when the person is nearby; credit cards and other magnetically encoded cards are damaged or erased when in the pocket of someone experiencing this phenomenon.

Because all of these effects occur spontaneously, without any conscious control, replication in a research laboratory is challenging, if not impossible. The moods or states of mind that seem to provoke the effects most consistently are when the person is highly excited, mentally focused on a problem, agitated, stressed, or angry. Seemingly, when people abandon their normal brain function, they ignite an electrical charge that affords a new dimension in their abilities. This fully displays the electromagnetic creatures that we are. Diagnostic tools used by allopathic physicians actually monitor the electromagnetic frequencies of bodily organs and other systems.

One of the promising areas of research that may clarify how subtle currents and electrical frequencies govern biological and ecosystems is the remarkable findings about our capacity to perceive and unite with earth energies. Humans are interconnected with Earth's magnetic fields, and now there is proof that we are sensing it and, in part, reacting to these subtle currents. Stuart Gilder[213], a geophysicist at the Ludwig Maximilian University in Germany, says the work of Peter Hore, a physical chemist at Oxford, UK, needs to be expanded upon and refined so that eventually, biological science can begin utilizing a system of frequencies applied to correct specific disorders, both emotional and anatomical.[214]

More advanced technology that our medical team utilizes on our campus widely and thoroughly determines, using cellular resonance (electrical frequency), normal or abnormal states of health. Scientists at the top of their game, like Ulrich Henschke, a pioneer in the field of brachytherapy and student of Max Plack,[215] have pioneered ways to place isotopes into one's brain, observing and monitoring the subtle frequency currents that are neuronically moving through the pathways that create thoughts. These researchers' genius, woven together with artificial intelligence, have now discovered a way to predict thoughts and monitor them electronically. What this means for future advancements in attitudinal healing is endless! Once the inherent mental electric patterns have been established and scrutinized over time, it will be possible for the isotope therapy to begin to alter negative thoughts and quite possibly, even transfer them into positive thoughts. This means many brain disorders like low IQ, dyslexia, attention deficit disorder (ADD), and even autism will potentially be corrected. As promising as this is, there is an ethical concern that such therapy can be used in a manipulative and negative way.

Now, it is for us to determine how to channel this gift and utilize it in positive and effective ways for the progressive advancement of the mind and body.

Human Lightning Rods

Your odds of being struck by lightning are about the same as winning a state lottery. Yet, it's also true that people have won state lotteries multiple times, and lightning bolts have hit some on more than one occasion.

In Louis Proud's 2014 book *Strange Electromagnetic Dimensions*[216], he recounts the experiences of a U.S. Park Service ranger, Roy Sullivan[217], who was struck by lightning *eight times* and survived each electrifying encounter. The first strike occurred when he was a child cutting wheat in a meadow with a scythe. After he began his park ranger career in 1936, in Virginia's Shenandoah National Park, he was struck repeatedly over the years as if he had become a human lightning rod.

His injuries weren't life-threatening ---usually, his hair, eyebrows, and eyelashes would be singed or burned off. Not all the strikes happened while he was on ranger duty in the mountains. One strike was while he drove his truck, a second while he was in the front yard of his home, and a third took place as he fished alongside a pond. The last strike in 1977 left him with burns on his stomach and chest.

A statistics professor at George Washington University estimated that your chances of being struck by lightning as many times as Sullivan; work out to be one in many trillions--- 100 followed by 30 zeros. "It appears that when a person has been struck by lightning once, their chance of being struck by lightning again increases exponentially," concluded Proud in his book.

As with the street light phenomenon, being a target for the electromagnetic energy of lightning may involve a heightened physical state of conductivity. In coming chapters we'll examine how these states might be manipulated to achieve physical healing.

CHAPTER 12:

Three Healing 'Vibes': Loving-Kindness, Forgiveness & Gratitude

"The practice of forgiveness is our most important contribution to the healing of the world." - Marianne Williamson

Emotions are self-generated bio-electromagnetic frequencies that can ravage our minds and bodies if we choose to dwell on toxic feelings. Conversely, they can heal our minds and bodies if they are heartfelt, joyous proclamations.

Medical science has well-documented evidence that chronic stress and anger have negative effects on health and the human bio-electrical system.[218] Our body spews out supranormal levels of the stress hormone cortisol when our natural defense mechanisms are engaged. According to experts at The Mayo Clinic, cortisol "alters immune system responses and suppresses the digestive system, the reproductive system and growth processes."[219] The result of these alterations is a higher risk for heart disease, hypertension, and related cardiovascular disruption, cancer, sleep disturbances, weight gain, digestive problems and depression, to name just a few.

Opposingly, expressing love and compassion has direct health benefits.[220] Medical studies have thoroughly documented these phenomena over the past decade.

In my view, the three healing vibes of loving-kindness, forgiveness and gratitude provide more evidence of the bio-energy manipulation phenomenon as governed by our thoughts. These positive affirmations trigger the electrical release of hormone chemicals such as serotonin and dopamine with a healing potential that can be mentally directed anywhere in the system.

Hippocrates' psychotherapy team strives to help each of our guests to reach their maximum vista in affirmative thought. As a result of releasing their burdens, the participants in our program display remarkable improvements in their immune system function as reflected in their blood profiles. Although there needs to be more investigative research resulting in categorical and definitive science, I and the Institute are committed to positive thought as a central antidote to physical disorders.

Love Energy at the Heart of Healing

Studies clearly show that *social support*—connection and intimacy, or love—is a key factor (and in many cases, *the* key factor) in maintaining and achieving good health. Whether you're close to a spouse, a family member, a friend or a pet, there's something critically important about having supportive companions on your journey to health and healing.

A study in the journal *Brain, Behavior and Immunology* showed that a loving, supportive marriage increases the effectiveness of vaccines. A study conducted by a team of researchers at the University of Athens School of Medicine in Greece showed that a person's ability to express and receive love was the key factor in whether or not they got sick.[221]

Scientifically validated applications for healing with Love include Alzheimer's, arthritis, immune disorders, cancer, depression, diabetes, flu and other respiratory diseases, heart disease, high blood pressure, HIV/AIDS[222], insomnia, kidney disease, memory problems, overweight and obesity, pain (chronic), Parkinson's disease, post-traumatic stress disorder (PTSD), pregnancy problems, stress, stroke, and substance abuse.

The Loving-Kindness Technique

Loving-kindness originated in the religious traditions of Buddhism, Judaism, and Christianity, all of which described the concept as acts of kindness motivated by love.

In Buddhism, a loving-kindness meditation was developed to express this feeling toward self and others. This meditation form has been extensively studied for its therapeutic health benefits.[223] Research published in the journal *Brain & Behavior,* described how a science team used functional magnetic resonance imaging in 2014 to study the brains of volunteers engaged in a loving-kindness meditation. These volunteers engaged in directed well-wishing accompanied by silent repetition of the phrase, "may all beings be happy," to create a feeling of selfless love. This practice activated the blood-oxygen level-dependent signal in an area of the brain called the posterior cingulate cortex (PCC) and precuneus.[224] This area of the brain sends electrical signals to other parts of the brain and specific areas of the body to facilitate healing, as determined by a series of other experiments.

Among the findings:

i. An analysis of 20 randomized controlled trials of the meditative technique found it helpful in reducing symptoms of epilepsy, premenstrual syndrome, menopausal symptoms, mood and anxiety disorders, autoimmune illnesses, and the effects of neoplastic disease.[225]

ii. In this 8-week loving-kindness program study, 43 volunteers suffering from chronic low back pain were assigned to either a meditation group, or a standard care group. Post and follow-up analyses of both groups "showed significant improvements in pain" in the loving-kindness group, but no changes in the usual care group, according to the researchers.[226]

iii. Twenty-seven people who suffered two to ten migraine headaches a month, none of whom had ever meditated before, were put through 20-minute guided loving-kindness meditations during migraine episodes. Afterward, these volunteers reported an average 33% decrease in the severity of their pain symptoms.[227]

iv. Doing a loving-kindness meditation dramatically reduces high blood pressure by decreasing stress hormones. In turn, this practice helps to reduce cardiovascular disease risk factors. These were some of the findings from a 2015 study that evaluated a dozen volunteers, average age of 51 years, who did a 20-minute loving-kindness meditation practice.[228]

Exercising Forgiveness Helps to Heal You

It's important to understand that forgiving someone is for *your* sake, for *your* emotional healing, not to heal the person who you perceive has hurt you.

By holding onto resentments and grudges, it's easy to create problematic health consequences for yourself. Forgiveness is the choice you make to take responsibility for how *you* feel—the choice to experience a healing peace of mind and, with it, the removal of emotional barriers that impede wellness.

Larry Dossey[229], M.D., has been at the forefront of research on how the mind, using loving-kindness meditations and forgiveness, can exert healing effects on the body. His many books include *One Mind: How Our Individual Mind Is Part of a Greater Consciousness and Why It Matters*[230], *Healing Words: The Power of Prayer and the Practice of Medicine*[231], and *Healing Beyond the Body: Medicine and the Infinite Reach of the Mind*[232].

Fred Luskin[233], PhD, co-founder and director of the Stanford University Forgiveness Project[234] and author of *Forgive for Good: A Proven Prescription for Health and Happiness*[235], explains: "You have an unresolved grievance. You blame the person who hurt you for how bad you feel. Forgiveness is the peace you feel when you resolve that grievance."

Everyone can *learn* how to forgive. It's like tuning into a wavelength. "Forgiveness can be taught and learned, just like learning to throw a ball," observed researchers.

People who blame others for their troubles have a higher incidence of heart disease and cancer. Scientific studies also show that people who are forgiving have fewer health problems overall, including fewer physical symptoms from stress like high blood pressure and insomnia. One reason is that each time you revisit a sense of grievance, you inflict more stress on your body.

In a clinical study in which people imagined either forgiving or inversely not, those imagining forgiveness had increased blood flow, less muscle tension, and lower levels of stress hormones, while those not imagining forgiveness had negative changes in those measurements.

Forgiveness isn't about being a doormat for callous people or unjust situations. "Forgiveness doesn't mean condoning unkindness, forgetting that something painful happened, excusing poor behavior, or reconciling with the offender," Luskin says. "Forgiveness is a skill that frees you from unnecessary emotional pain and poor health."

Imagine your mind as a television that gives you control to change the channel from feeling resentment to feeling forgiveness. In order for you to tune in to The Forgiveness Channel: Let go.

- Look for people—possibly members of your own family—who have forgiven others. Ask them to tell you their stories to motivate you to follow a similar path.

- Recall times in the past when you have forgiven someone. How did you feel afterward? Did the release of that burden in any way help to rejuvenate your health or sense of well-being?

- Get inspiration from people who have grown beyond having a desire for resentment and revenge. Read books like A Man Named Dave: A Story of Triumph and Forgiveness (about a man who suffered child abuse and subsequently forgave his father) and A Human Being Died That Night: A South African Story of Forgiveness (which recounts how the families of apartheids victims went about forgiving those who had tortured and killed their loved ones.)

- Practice forgiving small offenses. For example, forgive a driver who cuts you off in traffic. You can also forgive a friend who didn't call when she or he said they would.

- Remind yourself of times when you hurt others and needed their forgiveness. How did you feel when they forgave you? What did that feeling inspire you to do in return?

  - Notice when someone is kind to you even after you've been hurtful.

  - Observe and note how often you naturally forgive those you love.

125

A Positive Emotion Refocusing Technique

Maintaining peace in any situation—no matter how disturbing—is necessary to facilitate forgiveness, says Dr. Luskin. He has developed a technique called PERT: Positive Emotion Refocusing Technique[236]. "It can help counteract the effects of an unresolved grievance or ongoing relationship problem," he says. It consists of two steps:

1. Bring your attention fully to your abdomen and inhale deeply one or two times. As you inhale, gentle push your belly out. As you exhale, consciously relax and "soften" your belly.

2. Take a third deep breath and imagine someone you love or a beautiful scene in nature that fills you with awe. While continuing with your abdominal breathing, ask the peaceful part of you what you can do to resolve the difficulty.

Health Conditions That Forgiveness Helps To Treat

Alcoholism, Anxiety, Cancer, Cardiovascular Disease, Depression, Drug Addiction, High Blood Pressure, pain, stress, and wounds.

Medical Study Examples:

- Exercising forgiveness lowers blood pressure and heart rate and has other "beneficial effects for the forgiver's health."[237]

- In a study of 99 people with cardiovascular disease, forgiveness was found to accelerate recovery. "Forgiveness may impact cardiovascular health not through a myocardial or vascular pathway, but through another as yet unidentified mechanism."[238]

- University of Tennessee psychologists used 81 adults to assess the health benefits of exercising forgiveness. There were five measures of health—physical symptoms, medications used, sleep quality, fatigue, and somatic complaints—all showed improvements from a forgiveness exercise.[239]

- A total of 61 patients with chronic low back pain were evaluated for forgiveness-related variables. Those who were able to forgive others and perceived transgressions experienced lower pain and less frequent lower back pain than those holding on to their anger and resentments.[240]

Expressing Gratitude Also Brings Healing

Alcoholism, anxiety, cancer, depression, high blood pressure, HIV/AIDS and chronic stress.

All of the above-mentioned maladies have been scientifically validated by applications of healing with assistance from Gratitude.[241]

"Gratitude is the feeling that you've received a benefit or gift provided by someone else—by another person, by God, by whatever source," said Robert A. Emmons, Ph.D.[242], a Professor of Psychology at the University of California at Davis, who has conducted studies on how gratefulness affects us emotionally and physically.

In one study, a group of people wrote down what they were grateful for, while another group wrote about what was going wrong in their lives. After a few weeks, those in the "gratitude group" had more energy and zest for life and slept better than those who were in the "pessimist group."

"An attitude of gratitude—even in the midst of suffering—is going to have a positive effect on the health of the body and mind," he says. "Being grateful builds social relationships, for example, and studies show that people with more social support are healthier than those without it."

Can you *develop* an attitude of gratitude? Yes, says Dr. Emmons. It is not a trait but a conscious choice. "Gratitude can be cultivated," he says. In this section, he and other experts show you how to do just that.

For example, a series of three studies conducted by psychologists for the Journal of Personality and Social Psychology examined the effects of gratitude on people with neuromuscular disease. Compared to the control group, which didn't make a daily practice of expressing gratitude, those with gratefulness exhibited a heightened well-being in nearly all of the outcome measures. This resulted in physical and emotional benefits, which improved their overall health and coping behaviors.[243]

Additionally, at the Institute of HeartMath in Boulder Creek, Ca., Dr. Rollin McCraty & Dr. Glen Rein have conducted research that shows love as a real concept in healing. This emotion has measurable physiological effects, even at the DNA level.[244]

Rein and McCraty and their colleagues are hypothesizing a new system of communication in the body. It's an energy-field system that they refer to as 'cardioneuroimmunology',[245] which occurs as a coherent energy pattern of the heart center, during the feeling and expression of love, influencing energetic events in the body. As one example of their research, they found fifty-thousand receptor sites on the heart that directly communicated with Brain function.

CHAPTER 13:

Practices and Technologies for Bio-frequency Healing

Everything is energy, and that's all there is to it. Match the frequency of the reality you want and you cannot help but get that reality. It can be no other way. This is not philosophy. This is physics."- Albert Einstein.

Imagine a world where bio-medical devices could predict or diagnose your chances for acquiring a disease—and then reduce or eliminate your risk before the malady could emerge and damage your health. Today, we are already living in this world with rings that measure our sleep patterns, watches that measure our heart rate, aerobics, and phones that act as on-the-spot cardio measurement devices.

Earlier in this book, we highlighted current technology that is expeditiously advancing. Cyberscan[246], Biowell[247], and the Aura Meter are just a few examples of this quantum leap in science. The Cyberscan can map the patterns of energy that precede and cause physical, emotional, and psychological diseases. It can also prescribe the most healing approach for each person and validate the effectiveness of the actual practitioner working with the patient.

As in the Biowell, biofeedback biofrequency imaging reads a person's electronic signature and converts the data into color.

The Hunt Meter is based on the idea that human bioenergy fields oscillate at higher frequencies than EKG or EEG machines can measure; Dr. Hunt developed a high-frequency instrument to measure the bioelectrical energy radiating from the body's surface, which gives off frequencies 1000 times faster than any other electrical activity of the body. Dr. Hunt's Bioenergy Fields Monitor[248] is a high-frequency, low amplitude system with sensitive, low subtle energy optic lead cables.

Biofeedback is Important to the Field of Self-Healing

Studies of biofeedback have shown that physical processes thought to be autonomous could be brought under conscious control. One example is with Gregorian chants, where humming, singing, and whistling all create energy to perk up a person's emotions and bring on expanded states of consciousness.[249] Study results also indicate that we can learn to direct our own immune and endocrine systems using conscious intention. That means we need to find the mind practice most conducive to us as individuals for the development of this self-healing potential.

Solfeggio Frequencies

It has been said that our oldest human ancestors did not speak but communicated by banging on the head of a drum that created a resonance note that they learned to interpret. As evolution unfolded a wide variety of frequencies were gathered together into the form of instruments. Some percussion others wind instruments, some strings and eventually harpsichord and piano.

All of these sounds were harvested from earth's abundance residing in nature. Like parrots we began to capture these frequencies and create scales that mimicked them. As we know, a beating drum provokes energy within our cells and muscles that engage movement and dance. This gathering reaches our primal brain unlocking biological expression as we move up the scale of these sounds (frequencies), they touch our heart, our mind, consciousness and souls. I suppose that all of this was created over millennia as a healing tone to bring about balance and glee for ailing personas.

This gathering of instrumental splendor until the mid-twentieth century contained what is known as solfeggio frequencies[250].

There are seven:

- **360 HZ** - Is known to liberate one from fear and guilt.
- **417 HZ** - Helps in facilitating change including reversing untenable situations.
- **528 HZ** - To manifest miracles and transformation including genetic DNA repair.
- **639 HZ** - To improve and bond relationships and attract reconnection.
- **741 HZ** - To foster solutions and provoke self-expression.
- **852 HZ** - Spiritual realignment.
- **963 HZ** - For self-realization and relationship unity.

It is remarkable and exciting to consider that our forebears were so attuned to their environment and the universe in which they resided that they captured energy, refined it into notes, and manifested instruments they created and played. Musicality is today considered entertainment. Not long ago, physicians, as healers, used sound frequencies as a core prescription.[251]

Here at Hippocrates, we have been using sound healing for 7-decades and observing how it assists in degrading layers of emotional prohibition so that true self-expression can be achieved on a physical and psychological basis.

Somehow, in 1955, a worldwide agreement was signed where the signatories declared that the middle "A" be forevermore tuned to exactly 440 HZ. This frequency became the standard ISO -16[252] Reference for tuning all musical instruments based on a chromatic scale which is employed worldwide and was born out of western dogma. All of the other notes are tuned to standard mathematical ratios leading to and from 440 HZ. This is why a piano tuned in Florida is the same as in London, and it is the same as in China. From that moment forward, the healing frequencies that endless generations bathed themselves in were squashed.

Classical music, for example, by someone like Mozart, who used the original keyboards, sounds significantly different today than it would have at the time he composed it. Remarkably, composers and musicians were part of the healing arts, and now they are part of the entertainment industry.

As recent as 1986, Japanese scientist Susumu Ohno authenticated that notes affected nucleotides within your bodily systems[253]

Notes	Nucleotides
A	G
C	T
G	C
D	A

This has been verified scientifically but is especially visually easy to see when you begin applying these notes/frequencies to structure since sound moves matter. The term that is used is cymatics[254]. You may want to access some of the photographs when these healing frequencies are applied to sand and water. When you go back in history, many of the original advanced cultures produced art that mimicked these patterns. This is vivid proof that they had a grasp that seems absent today. When applying the Solfeggio frequencies previously mentioned, the soundwaves enhance healthy cellular growth and activate neurotransmitters and hormones that connect brain function to consciousness.

We are entering a new frontier that was breached before by our conscious primal ancestors and we must humble ourselves and recognize the powerful subtleties that are waiting for us to tap into them in the quest to become whole again. Crawl back into the womb of nature and the abundance it offers to be reborn into the Quantum world that seeks peace, healing, and unity, this will be yours.

Hypnosis Can Orchestrate Healing Effects in the Body

Hypnosis has been used as anesthesia in surgery since the 19th century. These surgeries using hypnosis range from fractures and dislocations to vaginal hysterectomies and heart surgeries. One dental surgeon successfully stopped his patient's bleeding in 75 hemophiliacs using hypnotic suggestion. Asthma has been alleviated using self-hypnosis.[255] Perhaps the most remarkable use of hypnosis has been the enlargement of women's breasts, the most convincing study being one in which 70 women experienced an average bust increase of nearly two inches, and some three inches and more, from imagery and suggestions made in trance to stimulate blood flow into that part of their bodies.[256]

Many studies show that hypnosis – both induced by a hypnotist or self-induced - can greatly accelerate one's recovery from injuries, illness, or disease. Here are a few examples:

- *The American Journal of Clinical Hypnosis* published a study in 1983 showing that "hypnosis facilitated dramatic enhancement of burn wound healing" in all test patients.[267]
- A study of 185 women by a science team in Israel and presented in 2004 to the European Society of Human Reproduction, found a pregnancy rate among women who were hypnotized when transplanted with embryos was more than twice that of women given transplants without hypnosis.[268]

Imagery and Visualization Enhances Health

Using the mind's power of visualization to evoke a positive wellness response is a practice woven into the fabric of the healing rituals used by many ancient cultures. Today, the Academy for Guided Imagery, led by a traditionally trained Ph.D. neuroscientist, instructs clinicians on how to use it with patients to lessen illness symptoms and enhance immune system functioning. Guided imagery is a practical, low-cost, easy-to-use tool for self-care, especially among cancer patients. A review by the American Cancer Society of 46 studies on imagery and cancer conducted from 1966 to 1998 revealed that guided imagery was effective in reducing pain, stress, depression, and other side effects associated with cancer treatment.

Studies have shown that interactive guided imagery can heal back pain associated with misaligned vertebrae. Dr. John Sarno's idea that back pain is the result of the mind's interference with nerve functioning and blood circulation will be described here, along with a case study testing the idea.

At the University of Arkansas College of Medicine, a team of researchers tested a 39-year-old woman who could use imagery to alter her immune system. She was verified as being able to change a positive chickenpox virus test into a negative and then back again to positive by simply imagining the virus growing and then eliminating it by sending visions of 'healing energy' to the affected areas of skin. This woman is using a technique known as guided imagery.[257] My work as director of the Hippocrates Health Institute has led me to widely employ attitudinal alterations in each and every individual that we work with. When effectively achieved over the decades we observed improvement with psychoneuroimmunology and other advanced techniques during psychotherapy sessions in both groups and individuals. Our comprehensive cancer program, which pioneering scientists lead, employs the most researched technique for altering cancer cell development with visualization or guided imagery.

One of my colleagues, the late Dr. Carl Simonton[258], conducted a famous series of guided imagery tests in which his patients were able to kill cancer cells by visualizing their shrinkage. Other studies have shown how negative mental states can depress the immune system and activate cancer cells.

A range of visualization and guided imagery techniques will be described here, along with their verification in tests done under laboratory conditions.

Meditation When Used with Visualization Creates a Healing Synergy

Experiments with heart patients found that meditation combined with visualization techniques caused overall cholesterol levels to drop[259] by 20 percent on average with angina attacks reduced[260] by 90 percent. These results demonstrate that the mind can have a positive impact on the physical causes of heart disease.

The Practice of Qigong

For a long time, this is how the National Qigong Association described this health maintenance practice: "Qigong is an ancient Chinese health care system that integrates physical postures, breathing techniques and focused intention. The word Qigong (Chi Kung) is made up of two Chinese words. Qi is pronounced *chee* and is usually translated to mean the life force or vital-energy that flows through all things in the universe. The second word, Gong, pronounced gung, means accomplishment, or skill that is cultivated through steady practice. Together, Qigong (Chi Kung) means cultivating energy, a system practiced for health maintenance, healing and increasing vitality.

For several decades, we have employed the ancient art and science of Qigong here at Hippocrates. One of our key faculty members achieved his doctorate in this masterful technique. An intentional movement that focuses on energy shifts that express and expand one's emotional and biological self empowers the body to remedy imbalance. There are hospitals in China that document recoveries from catastrophic diseases through the use of these powerful methods. On our campus, we observe the participant's release and reflection of self-realized acceptance. This motivational experience affords tools for healing at the cellular level.

The following case is documented in a 2004 science journal study article: A 58-year-old New Jersey man suffering from a series of chronic conditions, including high blood pressure, edema in the legs, asthma, a high prostate antigen level, and injuries from an auto accident, so he was put through a daily routine of four hours of qigong meditations combined with self-healing visualizations and guided imagery.

After ten sessions, he was able to discontinue all eight medications for his various ailments. His weight was down 35 pounds, the edema in his legs disappeared, his PSA level dropped from an 11 abnormal reading to 4, his blood pressure fell from 220/110 to 120/75, and he was healthy again.

The mystified authors of this study wrote: "This kind of simultaneous recovery from multiple conditions cannot be explained by any known medical theories.[261]

Major Breakthroughs in Regenerative Medicine

A study[262] published in April 2007 in the journal of *The Federation of American Societies for Experimental Biology,* reported the first part of what was described as "a major revolution in human regenerative medicine." The report identified how regenerative processes work by studying an evolutionary ancestor to humans. Sea squirts were the primary subjects researchers employed in unlocking the powers of tissue regeneration. When a sea quirt's physical limb was missing, what remained was the invisible electromagnetic blueprint. RNA and DNA surrounded this field, manifesting tissue that replaced the missing appendage.

Principles behind the processes of self-healing and organ regeneration were described for the first time. This will enable humans to one day regenerate hearts, missing limbs, and other body parts using gene therapy.

Findings from the bio-energy field that show effects at the genetic and cellular levels from regenerative processes associated with energy practitioners, spontaneous remission, and the placebo effect give us hope that regenerative medicine is on the verge of tremendous breakthroughs.

Energy Techniques Already in Practical Use

Understanding how 'energy medicine' works in theory needs to begin with describing the multiple ways it already operates in practice.

We need to start with acupuncture, a practice with at least 2,500 years of trial-and-error development culminating in relatively recent scientific documentation of its healing effects.

Acupuncture is a technique that was ridiculed by Western science and medicine through most of the 20th century, often labeled a 'ridiculous pseudoscience'. After hundreds of peer-reviewed medical journal studies, acupuncture has now been accepted by the National Institutes of Health and other government organizations around the world as providing "clear evidence" for a wide variety of effective treatments for diseases and health problems.

A 2005 study published in *The Lancet,* for instance, tested 294 osteoarthritis patients and concluded that acupuncture reduced their knee pain.[263]

A Mayo Clinic study of 50 fibromyalgia patients in 2006 found joint stiffness, muscle pain and fatigue to be greatly reduced from acupuncture treatment. [264]

In a 2005 study published in *Obstetrics & Gynecology,* a group of 85 women experienced a one-third reduction in bladder control problems after sessions with acupuncture.[265]

The list of studies of ailments showing the benefits of acupuncture goes on and on, ranging from stroke rehabilitation to menstrual cramps, stress reduction, carpal tunnel syndrome, and post-surgical pain.

Archaeological speculation has been that slivers of bone constituted the first acupuncture needles in China several thousand years ago, later replaced by bronze, silver, or gold needles. The numbers and locations of specific acupuncture sites on the human body have also evolved. Originally, there were thought to be 365 pressure points used on the anatomy, one for each day of the year. As more pressure points were added over the centuries, that number eventually grew to more than 2,000 needle sites being utilized today.

How do needles and pressure points affect biology and produce such a wide array of healing activity? Is acupuncture really a manipulation of the bio-energy field?

Beyond speculating that the pressure points stimulate the central nervous system to release neurotransmitters and hormones, conventional Western-trained scientists are mostly unable to explain how acupuncture produces its healing effects within their rigid biological standards.

At least four general biological responses have emerged and been acknowledged by the National Institutes of Health as having been confirmed by medical science studies examining acupuncture's effects on the human body:

1. Acupuncture releases opioid peptides to exert analgesic effects and reduce physical pain.

2. Both the pituitary gland and the hypothalamus are stimulated by acupuncture resulting in other systemic effects.

3. Use of acupuncture affects neurotransmitters and neurohormones, as well as the regulation of blood flow.

4. Immune system functions are enhanced by the use of acupuncture.

Functional magnetic resonance imaging (fMRI) of acupuncture effects in the human brain, as performed at Harvard Medical School and elsewhere, showed that areas of the brain involved in pain sensation and processing undergo dramatically decreased activity when pressure points are probed, simultaneously releasing hormones and enhancing immune cell functions.

A key question emerging from this early research was whether all acupuncture points on the body exert similar effects on the brain and on body functions or do the individual points really correspond to specific brain areas and body functions, as the acupuncture tradition claims. Skeptics believed the entire range of effects seen with acupuncture could be due to the placebo effect, the power of belief to activate body functions.

To answer that question, along with the placebo-related doubts posed by persons with limited thinking, subsequent research examined acupoint-specific fMRI patterns in the brain by having volunteers experience both real and staged acupuncture procedures. A 2005 study, for instance, found that actual acupuncture at specific points causes "specific and largely predictable areas of brain activation and deactivation"[266] In the meridian (the body's electric network), the acupuncture needle is applied, relating to specific organs that, in fact, are reflected in the brain.

A 2010 meta-analysis (comparative evaluation) of 34 studies done using fMRI to investigate the effects of acupuncture on the cerebral cortex concluded that "most studies suggest that acupuncture can modulate the activity within specific brain areas."[267]

Even more intensive studies followed. Published in the journal *Evidence Based Complementary Alternative Medicine* in 2014, a study placed the focus on using fMRI to observe brain areas activated by the use of acupuncture on one specific body area—the Taichung (LR3) acupoint, an important site in acupuncture tradition, located on the top of the foot in the depression at the junction of the 1st and 2nd metatarsal bones. This point is related to the liver, head, and eyes in the science of traditional acupuncture.

With 15 volunteers, both acupuncture and a fabricated acupuncture procedure were used in this experiment as they were monitored using fMRI; the volunteers didn't know whether they had received the real or placebo treatment when needles were applied. True acupuncture was done at this body site (but not the staged procedure) activating brain areas related to vision, movement, sensation, emotion, and analgesia. This experiment confirmed "that meridians and points (LR3) exert effects on specific brain areas," reported the research team. Equally important, the placebo effect played no role in activating these brain areas.[268]

Mainstream Western medicine still finds it difficult to accept how practices like acupuncture, acupressure, and qigong work. Ironically, the father of Western medicine, Hippocrates, employed his own form of acupuncture. Debate continues to rage over exactly what this 'life force' energy is and why it doesn't fit neatly into conventional scientific explanations for how biological systems function. It would behoove the academic and medical community to study the history and roots of their modern allopathic methods.

For too long, most of Western allopathy has remained skeptical of energy medicine "because no anatomical structures were known that might support Eastern theories of energy lines traversing the body," wrote Daniel J. Benor, M.D., in his book *Consciousness Bioenergy and Healing*. "The meridians do not correspond in any way to the well-mapped peripheral or autonomic nervous system, and until recently, no other communication network in the body had demonstrated that it could support such theories."[269]

James Oschman[270] has proposed that "the act of puncturing the skin with an acupuncture needle simulates an injury and thereby elicits the local and systemic cascade of regulatory, restorative, repair, and regenerative processes associated with wound healing."[271]

Chinese medicine is based on the concept of Qi, or life energies within the body "which interact with and resonate with those of the environment and of the worlds of spirit...Chinese medicine also views the body holistically, assuming that a part will reflect the whole...if the physical and/or energetic body are holograms, this would help to explain how acupuncture diagnosis can be based on the appearance of the tongue or condition of the teeth, and how treatments may be applied to points on the ear, hand, or foot that correspond to each of the various organs."

Hippocrates Institute has offered acupuncture, acupressure, and acupoint therapy since our inception. In addition, Tai Chi and Qigong have been tools that we have successfully employed. Clinically, we have observed a consistent phenomenon where a person's problems are expeditiously dealt with when the electro-magnetic fields of the meridian circuitry are stimulated and engaged. Think of the disorder as a clogged pipe and the acupuncture/pressure as the high-speed laser that removes the blockage. Another perspective is offered by Richard Gerber, M.D., author of *Vibrational Medicine: The Handbook of Subtle-Energy Therapies.* "The acupuncture meridians are the conduits of energy flow that make up this subtle energetic network. It has been demonstrated that the electrical characteristics of the meridians, as measured through the acupoints, contain important information about the status of the body's internal organs. The subtle energies flowing through the meridians are not electrical in nature, but they are able to induce electrical fields and currents because of their magnetic properties. This energy, known to the Chinese as chi, is actually a manifestation of the life force which animates and energizes living systems."

Acupressure Also Triggers the Energetic System

The healing picture that acupuncture presents us is complicated by the fact that Chinese, Japanese and Korean traditions sometimes differ concerning which of the 2,000 Qi points should be used, though they seem in agreement about many of the key central points. Additionally, Japanese acupuncturists use shorter and thinner needles than their Chinese counterparts, and in the Japanese tradition, these needles hardly pierce the skin.

We must also keep in mind that the use of needles isn't the only way that acupoints are stimulated and Qi energy is released. Applying finger pressure (acupressure) to acupoints and meridians can be effective, so can electroacupuncture (sending electrical currents into the acupoints) or sonopuncture (applying sound waves to the acupuncture points.) Even cupping heated jars over acupoints or burning an herb called moxa over the body areas can provide adequate stimulation, according to researchers who have studied these various techniques.[272]

How can we reconcile all of this seeming confusion? First, we have to acknowledge that a lot more research still needs to be done. Mapping the meridians and the specific brain functions activated by acupoint stimulation remains a dynamic research exploration.

From what we already know about energy systems in general and how they may operate, it shouldn't be surprising or confusing that the flow can be manipulated and directed by any kind of trigger, be it a needle or finger pressure, heat or sound that stimulates and calibrates a heightened body energy flow. Advanced sound in vibrational technologies are also employed on these meridians with great success.

Electric Food Therapy

In addition to traditional therapies, our foundational energy provider is nutrition. Anatomically, we are flesh and bone. Yet, what governs their existence is electrical frequency. We share this planet with eight million other species who are also electric creatures. Every one of them, in their natural setting, consumes only raw, uncooked foods. Humans are the only species that choose to cook, process, chemicalize, irradiate, and preserve what we swallow.

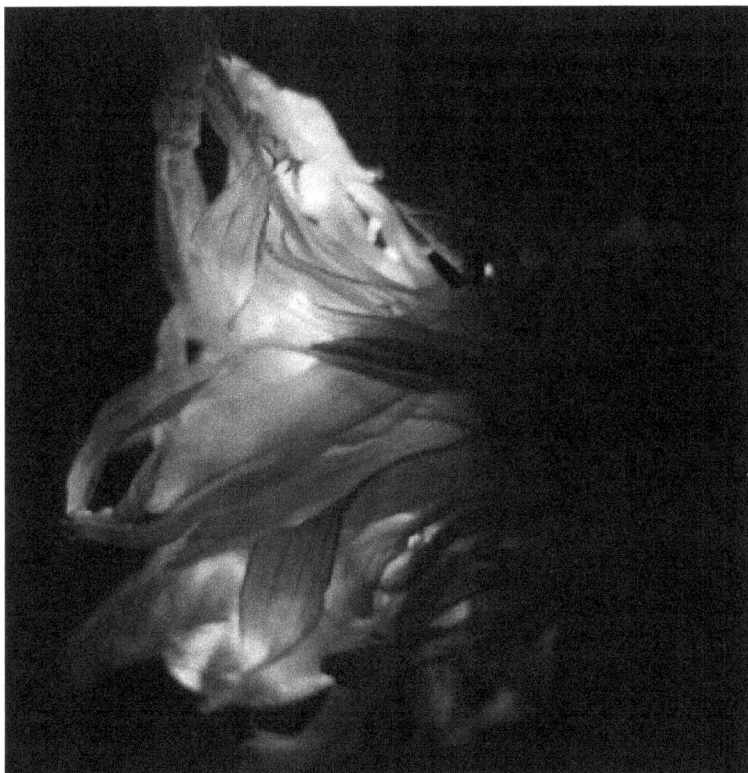

There is no longer a legitimate debate on the original diet that humans embraced. Anthropologist Dr. Richard Leakey[273] discovered this after looking at thousands of teeth specimens from pre-homo sapiens to the present day. From the indentations on the molars, it is clear that we consumed only plant-based fare.[274] We were not hunters and gatherers but nomads and gatherers. Cooking came long after the original people emerged from a valley in Ethiopia. Uncooked plants without animal food consumption is today called a Raw Vegan diet. It is bountiful in all of the essential nutrients, but most importantly, it affords the necessary electrical charge for filling the body's needs in all biological systems.

When we feed our physiology with electrical nutrition and our emotional persona with high-frequency food, we not only sustain life but thrive. Our research has shown that the increased amplitude harvested from fresh, raw plants that are immediately consumed places a virtual shield around our cells, protecting us from free radical damage. This damage has been noted since Dr. Harman's discovery at the University of Nebraska. He found free radicals to be the cause of all premature aging and disease.[275][276]

Emotional Freedom Technique

When people are making a transition to veganism or a raw living foods diet, they are sometimes haunted by the ghosts of their previous toxic eating habits. That dietary haunting often comes in the form of food cravings generated by withdrawal from the addictive grip of sugar, fats, salt, and void (or empty) carbohydrates.

Many of the therapeutic strategies used to control noxious food cravings begin with reducing the levels of stress that often trigger these cravings. Findings from medical science studies have elevated one approach over most others in its ability to defuse stress and control cravings---it's called the Emotional Freedom Technique[277], and it's based on the human energy field!

A member of the energy therapies family which includes acupuncture, acupressure, and shiatsu, the Emotional Freedom Technique (EFT) was designed to be used in a therapeutic setting to reduce stress and painful emotions associated with psychological trauma, poor health conditions, and toxic thoughts. This technique makes use of the human body's energy field—the 'meridians', as ancient Chinese medicine refers to it. This assists in the removal of many psychological obstacles to health and healing.

A clinical psychologist, Dr. Roger Callahan[278], a professor at Eastern Michigan University, was seeking a simple technique to heal people from stress-related disorders such as those caused by trauma and phobias, along with food cravings and other toxic compulsions. He studied traditional Chinese acupuncture and its 'meridian' points during the 1980s and, from that, developed a system of algorithms using a sequence of finger tapping along these energy field meridian points, rather than using acupuncture needles, to help heal psychologically-based ailments. He called the technique Thought Field Therapy, and it remains cutting edge in the field of psychological science and treatment.

According to the Thought Field Therapy's website,[279] this technique spawned a range of imitators and innovators. The most significant may have been developed by Stanford-trained engineer Gary Craig in the 1990s. His technique simplified the practice. He released a program that was a clear, simple approach to the utilization of this proven technique. Craig's training video, is called the EFT (Emotional Freedom Therapy) Course. Craig's system and related research are available on his website: https://www.palaceofpossibilities.com/.

This EFT approach soon became a centerpiece of the 'energy psychology' field. As a review published in a 2008 issue of the journal *Psychotherapy* observed: "Energy psychology has reached the minimum threshold for being designated as an evidence-based treatment, with one form having met the APA (American Psychological Association) criteria as a 'probable efficacious treatment' for specific phobias and weight loss." [280]

An overview of how the technique works in practice was provided by Nick Ortner, author of the 2013 book *The Tapping Solution*. "We literally tap with our fingertips on our body's meridian points while we mentally focus on our issue, whatever it is, such as the craving for sugar. The technique sends a calming signal to that part of our brain called the amygdala, which is responsible for our stress responses."[281]

Described below is how you can utilize this helpful technique.

Normally, with EFT, you begin by thinking about the problem or craving, visualize it, and feel it in your body. Then do the tapping on the energy pressure points as you repeat an affirmation to yourself, such as 'Even though I have this craving for sugar, I accept myself," That is a very simplified version of the practice, very much a mind/body sort of practice, and you can learn more in detail by accessing www.eft-help.com.

Numerous medical studies of EFT have been completed, many of them gauging its effectiveness in taming food cravings and the extent of subsequent weight loss. For example, psychologists in Australia put 96 overweight or obese adults through a four-week training in EFT to test the reduction in food cravings. (Chocolate cravings were most commonly chosen as a target by the volunteers). The majority of the participants were women over 40 years of age. Their progress was assessed at 6-month and 12-month intervals. The study results were clear and as the authors summarized it: "Significant improvements occurred in weight, body mass index, food cravings, subjective power of food, craving restraint, and psychological coping."[282][283]

There is a range of peer-reviewed clinical research done on EFT and its energy field regulation for healing and health maintenance. These studies show positive results for the use of EFT in treating traumas, pain, mental disorders and food cravings, particularly in diminishing the cravings many people feel for addictive substances like sugar. [284]

- Significant improvements in measures of pain, depression, and anxiety became apparent when 59 veterans with clinical levels of post-traumatic stress disorder symptoms received six sessions of EFT. This led study researchers to conclude: "the ability of EFT to produce reliable and long-term gains after relatively brief interventions indicates its utility in reducing the estimated trillion-dollar cost of treating veterans in coming years."[285]

- Injured veterans with respiratory, immunological, and psychological problems were put through an 8-week EFT series of sessions, and the results were compared to a control group who received no intervention. Those who did EFT showed decreased somatic symptoms, lowered frequency and severity of respiratory symptoms, increased lymphocyte proliferation (a strengthened immune system), and overall improved health and quality of life.[286]

- Twenty-two students suffering from a range of phobias completed five two-minute rounds of EFT treatment intervention. Three tests were administered afterward, measuring behavior, distress, and anxiety. In all three measures, the students completing EFT showed marked improvement, findings which confirmed previous studies on using EFT to treat specific phobias.[284]

So, how does EFT work physiologically? How can thoughts and actions together trigger an energy field response to bring about measurable and beneficial physical and mental changes? Evidence is still catching up to theory and practice.

Our Hippocrates programs have employed a wide array of mind-altering and habit-breaking processes and methods for 7-decades. Our 2023 book, "**Self-Healing Diet**,"[288] explores many of the clinical findings revealed by the use of these tools, which require discipline but often can be achieved alone without doctors, therapists, and other professionals.

Brain neuroimaging researchers at Harvard Medical School documented how stimulating the acupressure points, as happens with EFT, decreases arousal in the amygdala section of the brain as if a dimmer switch had been activated. The analogy to an electrical system is quite appropriate.

This brain area gets stimulated when you feel negative emotions or stress; it's also activated by food cues, such as smells or visual stimuli, which can produce toxic food cravings. Acupressure point stimulation deactivates portions of the amygdala brain area so food cues don't get activated as quickly or as easily.[289][290]

As further elaboration on the neurobiological basis for how this happens, New York Internist Ronald A. Ruden, M.D., prepared a research paper[291] in 2005 offering the view that tapping "causes a generalized release of serotonin via ascending pathways" and that, combined with the release of targeted emotions from visualization, triggers glutamate "in areas corresponding to the neural circuit that initially encoded the conditioned fear." This multi-sensory stimulation "affects the entire brain including the amygdala and prefrontal cortex." Where the tapping on the body occurs, and depending on the intensity of the tapping, affects the brain's serotonin system.[292] How this works is that it creates a chemical cascade reducing stress and further releasing glutamate.

To simplify, what we are talking about here is an electrochemical process that involves brain hormones like serotonin, the calcium ion, and a physical energy field within and around the body with pathways (meridians) that can be mapped. Joaquin Andrade, M.D. and David Feinstein, Ph.D., wrote "that the body is surrounded and permeated by an energy field which carries information. Disturbances in this energy field are said to be reflected in emotional disturbances."[293] This is still a controversial idea in psychotherapy. Yet, there has been research on the subject for years.

Research authors reported back in 2004, "The concept of energy fields carrying information that impacts biological and psychological functioning is appearing independently in the writings of scientists from numerous disciplines, ranging from neurology to anesthesiology, from physics to engineering, and from physiology to medicine. In energy psychology, this two-part formulation, in which biochemistry and invisible physical fields are believed to be working in tandem, has been used to explain the rapid changes that are often witnessed in long-standing emotional patterns. Changes in the energy field are understood as having the power to shift the organization of electrochemical processes. Many of the electrochemical processes that are probably involved have been mapped. One hypothesis is that the signal sent by tapping collides with the signal produced by thinking about the problem, introducing noise into the emotional process, which alters its nature and its capacity to produce symptoms. Enhanced serotonin secretion also correlates with tapping specific points."[294]

Another clue about what is happening in the body with tapping concerns the mechanoreceptors. They are scattered throughout the human body, but centralized in certain locations corresponding to acupressure points. These are specialized receptors (free nerve endings) sensitive to stimulation, such as tapping and massage, on the skin surface. Somatic pressure releases emotions stored in the body. Signals initiated by tapping go directly to the brain and to those brain areas where an emotional problem has its neurological roots. This signal disrupts the already established patterns, which drive disordered thinking and resulting toxic behaviors. Such a biological harboring of emotions is often called 'cellular memory.'

Professor Raphael Mechoulam, in the early 1960s, discovered a systemic system of receptor sites strategically placed throughout the human anatomy. Today, this is known as a cannabinoid receptor site system. By 1964, he and his team employed plant-derived THC, and the first endocannabinoids were discovered in his advanced Israeli laboratory. We now know that one's mood, level of mental capacity, and outlook can be enhanced by utilizing cannabinoids to alter psychology. In addition, there is an ever-growing body of evidence that this system coordinates with immunity to provoke attacks against microbes and mutagens.

New Bio-Energy Technologies

Over the decades at Hippocrates, we have continued to add emerging technologies. These help us to rapidly increase bio-energy in our cells so that renewal and healing can occur expeditiously. Foundationally, an electrically charged diet of uncooked organic raw plant-based foods provides the core component in the body's ability to function at its highest level. Combining lifestyle and advanced technology, we have pioneered the field of progressive healthcare.

Just consider the fact that when a heart stops, we do not use chemistry to jumpstart it. We place two paddles on the chest that electrically shock the organ to once again reengage.

Mainstream medicine's diagnostic tools: MRI, Catscan, Ultra-sound, etc., are all measuring the subtle electric frequencies that propel all life, including the internal organs and skeletal system. In every cell, which as a gathering creates every organ and skeletal structure, there is a mathematically perfect connective process of communication and exchange. Allopathic and natural healthcare have struggled to help ailing humanity because they are working at a surface level with chemistry alone rather than dropping the veil and addressing the true essence of the body's frequency engine.

We employ noninvasive electromagnetic therapies such as Tesla, ONDAMED, Theragem, VIOFOR, H.R.V and Bio-well, H-Wave, Purewave and cold laser.

These are the cutting-edge tools of healthcare that will eventually replace the broken, matter-based biological systems that have universally been applied in the conquest of disease with questionable success.

Although electronic biofrequency therapies are advanced methods in helping to prevent and even remove disease, they are electric and require protection technologies so that the EMFs coming from the devices do not have any deleterious effect on your health. As a pioneer in this field, Hippocrates has collaborated and created EMF protection devices such as HHI 360 and HHI Pulse to do just that.

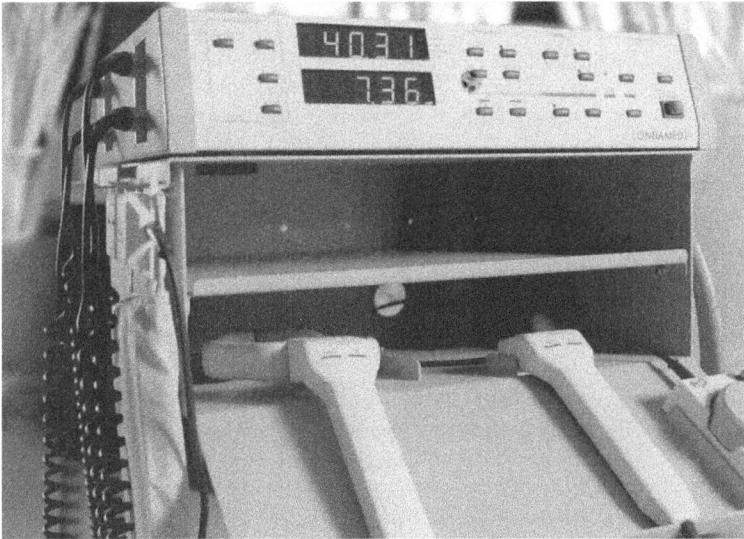

ONDAMED®

An electromagnetic frequency device that offers a highly specific biophysical analysis and application using focused electromagnetic waves. It's a combination of biofeedback and localized tissue stimulation. The practitioner rapidly scans the body's preferences, determines interference fields, and delivers the frequencies tailored to each individual. These healing micro-currents are able to penetrate deeply into ligaments, organs, and bone.

Reported benefits of ONDAMED® treatment include:

- Improvement in chronic pain
- Treatment of injuries and inflammation
- Improved blood circulation
- Activation of Lymphatic Drainage
- Increased cellular repair and regeneration
- Stimulation of detox and the release of toxins

During a session with this device, you may experience a mild tingling sensation or no sensation at all. Users commonly report feeling more relaxed and being able to think more clearly.

It can be used independently or in conjunction with any other treatment therapy. The device is registered with the U.S. Food and Drug Administration as a Biofeedback Class II medical device under the category of Neurology. In 2011 it was given Health Canada approval for treating wounds, soft tissue injuries and for general pain relief.

In her 2008 book, *Breakthrough: 8 Steps to Wellness*, the late actress Suzanne Somers, a cancer patient, had this to say about the system: "I now use the ONDAMED machine and the results have been truly miraculous. In just a short period of time I am no longer experiencing pain, swelling, or tenderness in the breast."

THERAGEM

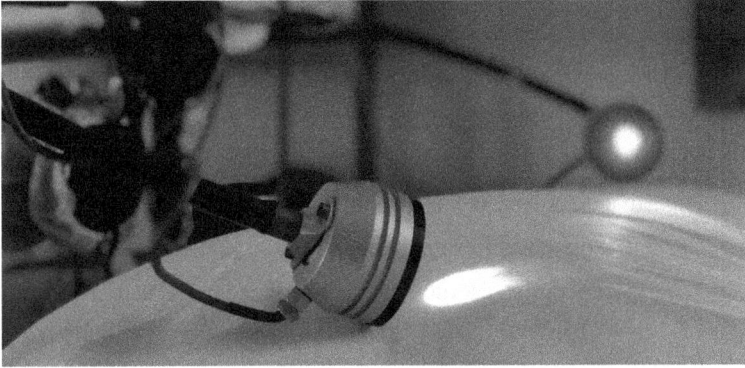

Theragem therapy is a cutting-edge fusion of gemstone and infrared technology. This advanced therapy combines the healing properties of precious and semi-precious gemstones with infrared light to promote healing, balance, and overall well-being. Sourced from a unique supplier in the United States, Theragem is used worldwide by healthcare and wellness practitioners as a gentle, non-invasive treatment to support the body's natural healing mechanisms.

Theragem therapy utilizes a sophisticated combination of full-spectrum light (chromatherapy) and gemstone energy. The system works by filtering colored light through carefully selected gemstones that resonate with the body's energy field. These gemstones, combined with gentle electromagnetic frequencies, harmonize the body and mind, addressing both physical and emotional imbalances.

The technology operates within the 600-900 nanometer range, known to influence the body's natural frequencies. Specifically, the 670 nm range, often called the "Wellness Zone," has been shown to help restore the body to a balanced and healthy state. Depending on the needs of the individual, different colors, gemstone types, and program settings are used to either energize sluggish areas or soothe overactive ones.

Theragem sessions typically last between 20 and 60 minutes. During this time, you will either sit or lie down while the Theragem lamps are directed at the targeted areas of your body. Participants often find the experience to be deeply relaxing, as the gentle warmth and energy from the gemstone-infused light work to balance the body. The specific combination of light and gemstones can be adjusted to provide either warming or cooling effects, depending on your body's needs at the time.

Theragem therapy is versatile and I have used it to address a wide variety of health conditions. These include, but are not limited to:

- Anxiety and depression
- Arthritis and joint pain
- Skin conditions like eczema and psoriasis
- Digestive disorders such as irritable bowel syndrome (IBS)
- Chronic fatigue and fibromyalgia
- Neurodegenerative disorders, including Alzheimer's and Parkinson's disease
- Respiratory issues such as asthma
- Stroke recovery, injury healing, and general anti-aging effects

For many people, improvements are felt within five to six sessions, with some acute conditions showing noticeable relief after just one or two visits. Chronic conditions may require more time to experience the benefits fully, but the overall improvement in energy, circulation, and muscle relaxation is evident throughout the therapy process.

By incorporating gemstone and infrared light, Theragem offers a holistic and natural approach to wellness. Through the synergy of light, color, and crystalline energy, this therapy serves as a powerful tool for restoring balance and supporting the body's inherent healing abilities.

COMRA

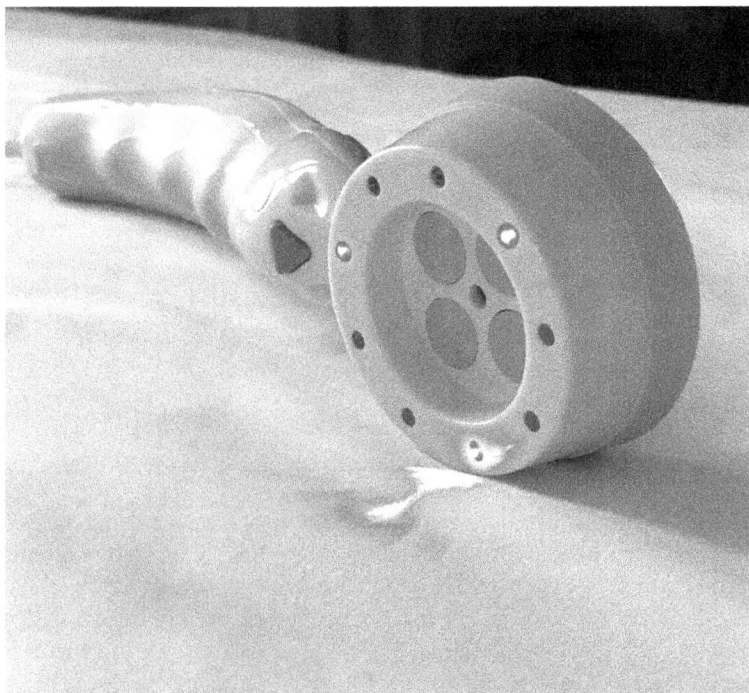

At Hippocrates, we also offer coMra therapy as part of our comprehensive approach to pain management and cellular regeneration. coMra, short for "coherence achieved through Modulation of different radiances," is a cutting-edge technology that combines laser, color, magnetism, and ultrasound to stimulate the body's natural healing abilities. Widely used by medical professionals around the world, coMra therapy offers a holistic and non-invasive treatment for a variety of conditions, with a particular focus on pain relief and tissue repair.

coMra therapy works by enhancing the natural regenerative processes of cells. The therapy's combined radiant properties create a harmonious effect that accelerates the repair of cell structures, boosts cellular energy metabolism, and regulates the body's internal processes. This coherent synergy between the different technologies is what makes coMra so effective. Whether addressing painful, inflamed areas or supporting the body through injury, stress, or disease, coMra helps cells heal faster and function more efficiently.

coMra therapy is particularly effective in treating chronic pain and difficult-to-manage conditions. Its wide range of applications includes:

- Back, joint, and arthritis pain
- Migraines and headaches
- Tissue repair and recovery from sports injuries
- Nerve repair, including neuropathy
- Inflammation and trauma
- Degenerative conditions like fibromyalgia and multiple sclerosis
- Respiratory issues such as sinusitis and asthma
- Circulatory and endocrine system support

In addition to pain relief, coMra therapy also offers broader health benefits. It can help restore vitality, boost immunity, and promote recovery from chronic illnesses and injuries. By supporting key systems like the central nervous, blood, and lymphatic systems, coMra aids in the body's overall well-being. It can also be used for detoxification, active aging treatments, and improving the function of internal organs.

Sessions with coMra therapy are non-invasive and relaxing. Depending on the severity of the condition, patients may notice improvements after just a few sessions, with chronic conditions requiring ongoing treatments to maintain results.

coMra's ability to treat a wide range of conditions while promoting cellular regeneration and pain relief makes it a unique and comprehensive solution for those seeking both immediate and long-term health benefits. Focusing on natural healing processes, coMra therapy helps restore balance and vitality to the body, offering a revolutionary approach to wellness that aligns perfectly with the holistic care I provide.

BrainTap

BEFORE

Spline-Map of Brain Electrical Activity

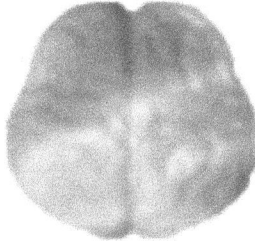

D = 40% (50 - 100%)

MIN  MAX

AFTER

Spline-Map of Brain Electrical Acivity

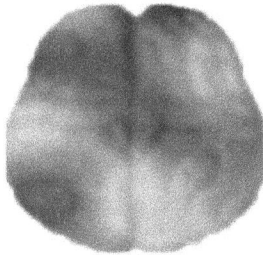

D = 88% (50 - 100%)

MIN  MAX

BrainTap Therapy is a non-invasive, drug-free method designed to relax, reboot, and revitalize your mind. This innovative therapy uses a combination of light and sound stimulation to guide your brain into a deeply relaxed state, often referred to as 'brainwave entrainment.' By aligning your brain's natural frequencies with specific stimuli, BrainTap Therapy helps you break free from stress, negative habits, and mental clutter while improving sleep, focus, and overall cognitive function.

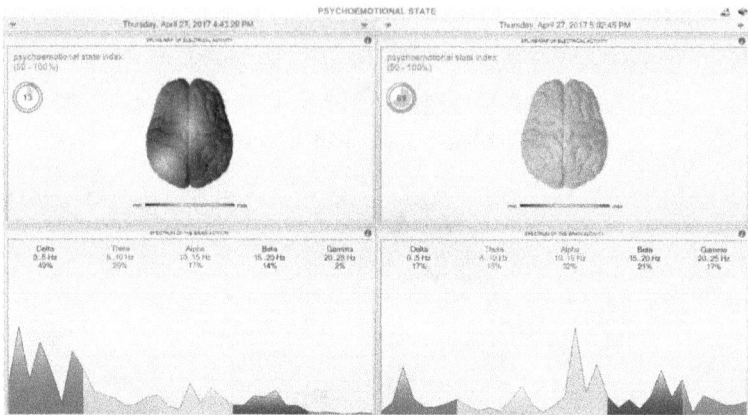

BrainTap Therapy operates through a specially designed headset that delivers gentle pulses of light and sound. These rhythmic pulses synchronize with your brain's natural wave patterns, creating a harmonious flow of brainwave activity. By guiding your brain into this state of deep relaxation, the therapy helps alleviate unwanted thought patterns, reduce stress, and promote mental clarity.

Whether you're seeking relief from anxiety, struggling with insomnia, or simply looking to enhance your mental performance, BrainTap Therapy offers a natural and effective solution. The therapy supports your brain's ability to achieve balance, leading to a more focused, calm, and productive state of mind.

Each BrainTap session is designed to be a calming and restorative experience. When you begin your session, you'll be seated in a quiet, comfortable space fitted with the BrainTap headset. As the session starts, gentle pulses of light and sound will gradually lead your brain into a state of deep relaxation. This sensation, known as brainwave entrainment, may evoke feelings of floating or a deep sense of calm – a natural response to the therapy's effect on your brainwaves.

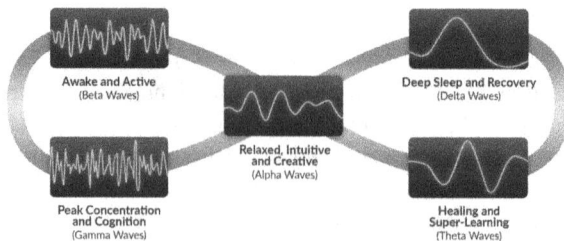

Awake and Active
(Beta Waves)

Deep Sleep and Recovery
(Delta Waves)

Relaxed, Intuitive and Creative
(Alpha Waves)

Peak Concentration and Cognition
(Gamma Waves)

Healing and Super-Learning
(Theta Waves)

From the BrainTap site Braintap.com

Sessions typically last between 15 and 30 minutes, during which you can fully relax and let the technology do its work. There's no need for conscious effort; allow yourself to be guided by the soothing rhythms of light and sound.

Regular BrainTap Therapy will help you:

- Improve your ability to fall asleep and stay asleep by training your brain to relax more efficiently.
- Clear mental fog, enhance concentration and improve memory with regular use.

Whether at work, in sports, or in daily life, BrainTap Therapy can help you perform at your peak by reducing stress and enhancing mental focus.

After your first session, it's common to feel a sense of mental clarity and refreshed alertness. Many of our guests report improvements in sleep, reduced stress levels, and an overall positive shift in mood. As each person's brain responds uniquely to the therapy, results may vary, but regular sessions are key to unlocking long-lasting benefits.

VIOFOR®

Viofor has subtle frequency projections that are electromagnetically stimulating to the body and aim to bring about homeostasis. This non-invasive technology taps into your electrical circuitry, recalibrating and adjusting the pulse that governs all bodily systems. Enhanced circulation and increased oxygenation to your tissues helps fight infection and strengthens your immune system.

The Bio-Well Scan®

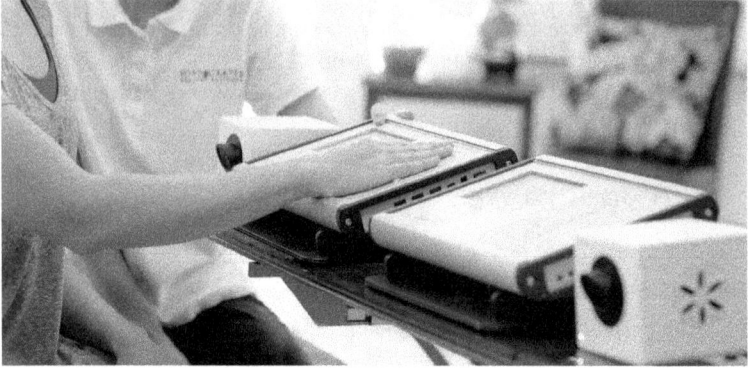

Bio-Well measures bio-markers from the human body's energy field as a general health observation tool, though it doesn't diagnose or treat any specific illness.

When guests arrive at our institute in West Palm Beach, Florida, they receive a scan on their first day to assess the stresses and strengths of their overall energy or 'life force' field. Measurements are taken from the fingertips of both hands using non-invasive photon emissions, and with special computer software, an image of their energy field is created and displayed to the participants in an easily understood picture and numerical format.

Developed by Konstantin Korotkov, a Professor of Physics at the St. Petersburg Federal Research University of Information Technologies, the device helps to guide our health care professionals in collaborating with our guests to design the foremost individualized and accurate health program for each person. Typically, after spending several weeks in our Life Transformation Program and continuing the lifestyle when they return home, subsequent bio-energy scans show a more uniform and vibrant energy field mirroring their overall improvement in well-being.

H-WAVE®

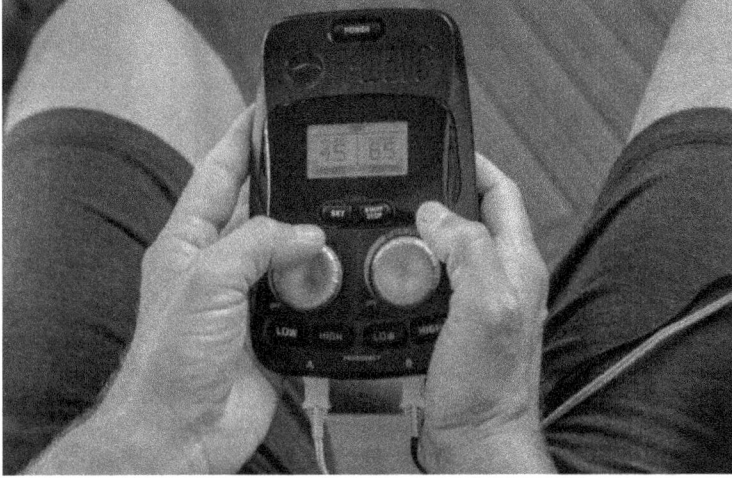

Our body has approximately sixty thousand miles of blood vessels. If you think that's impressive, consider that we have three times that distance (180,000 miles) of lymphatic vessels. "Viable" is considered to be the fundamental basis of all healthy tissue and all tissue healing. In order to achieve this dynamic balance, you have to enrich your body's plasma, increasing oxygen absorption, which helps to purge the tired and worn-out cells.

This physiological function is called "fluid dynamics." It is naturally achieved when blood consistently flows in the desired direction to carry away debris and bring new, life-renewing cells.

So, what does H-Wave® have to do with "fluid dynamics"? Absolutely everything! The core function of H-Wave® is the facilitation of fluid dynamics. This energetic exchange of charged interstitial fluids will help to achieve equilibrium, as described above.

H-Wave® uses technology that is patented, trademarked, and uniquely different than all other electronic waveforms. H-Wave® helps to facilitate a "harmonious" (no tetany or spasm) muscle contraction, which is the primary physiologic catalyst for increased circulation and lymphatic drainage. The increased blood flow from the force of a full cycle of "comprehensive" muscle contraction naturally provides the transportation to purge and rinse the tissues of metabolites, chemical irritants, and other toxic fluid pressures, using a lymphokinetic action.

A critical review of H-Wave® published in the Journal of Personalized Medicine stated that it increased blood flow by as much as 247% in the lower extremities and "has enough reasonable evidence to be considered" as a drug-free component of pain management treatment "given its excellent safety profile and relatively low cost." [295]

In our body, we have synapses. Synapses are similar in shape to a wishbone. They are how our cells communicate with each other, and they are like little spark plugs. Our synapses have a pre-synaptic area and a post-synaptic area. The space in between is called a synaptic cleft. Just like the spark from a spark plug ignites the combustion motor, the spark in the synaptic cleft ignites sensory and motor responses in the body.

H-Wave® so closely resembles this electrical spark or synaptic output that the body seems to recognize H-Wave® as inherently like its own electronic language and does not resist the signal. This represents a major breakthrough in electrotherapy and provides the "missing link" on how to get into the body without the body perceiving the waveform as a threat or enemy. This biomechanical action helps the body balance blood tissue chemistry through natural lymphokinetic fluid dynamics, slowing the pathogenic progression of many circulatory diseases while creating a homeostatic environment to enhance tissue regeneration and healing.

In essence, you may be able to reverse your symptoms and course of disease partially. These same fluid dynamics, in most cases, will significantly reduce acute or chronic pain for long periods of time by removing the "source or cause" of the pain signal. If there is no chemical irritation antagonizing the nerve, if there is no congestive pressure on the nerve, and if the nerve is able to get its proper uptake of oxygenated, nutrified blood flow, the opportunity for pain can be significantly minimized.

In the simplest terms, H-Wave® can profoundly increase blood circulation and lymphatic exchange to help you achieve a better quality of life.

QRS®

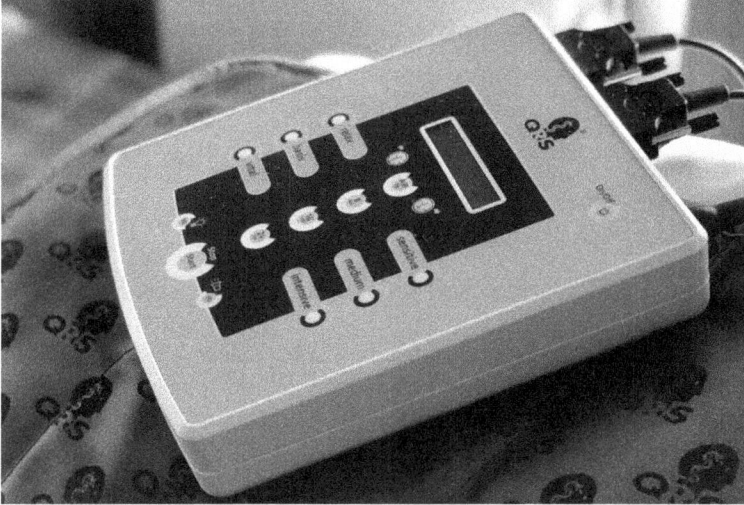

For seven decades we have been applying pulse therapies to help our participants recapture health and wellbeing. There is no bodily system that is not imbued with subtle electromagnetic currents. When these currents are supported to do their essential work, balance occurs. Disease is literally a blockage of normal currents and frequencies that manifest what we call disorder.

QRS (Quantron Resonance System) is a PEMF (Pulsed Electromagnetic Field). This advanced technology encompasses electromagnetic frequencies that resonate with naturally occurring rhythms of the human body. Your anatomy is made up of cells (approximately 40-100 trillion[296]). Each of these cells, when healthy, vibrates at a particular frequency. Microbes (bacteria and viruses), mutagens (growths and cancers), Lyme disease (spirochetes, etc.), heavy metals, pharmaceuticals and plastics, as well as chemicals and a continual bombardment of harmful renegade EMFs (Electromagnetic Fields) all distort cell normality. QRS projects harmonized fields of gentle electrical stimuli that assist the body's cells in regaining their power, therefore resisting disorder. Intercellular communication becomes normal again so that the body's multitude of pathways work the way they are meant to. Now and more so in the future, healthcare will increasingly rely on the electric language of skeletal and organ systems in the quest to maintain and regain health.

QRS is a central non-invasive tool in our repertoire. Every participant in our program is afforded many opportunities to utilize this state-of-the-art therapy.

Scalar Wave Protection®

SCWP is a recent technological advancement that amplifies the benefits of PEF (Pulsed Electromagnetic Field) therapy over a large geographical area; whereas QRS works on one person at a time, SCWP can pulsate in homes, buildings, and even over acreage. This technology was pioneered here at the Hippocrates and emits its powerful, protective frequencies throughout our sprawling campus.

Not only can it help attune one's bodily systems with geometrically sound subtle electromagnetic pulsations, but it can harmonize the environmental atmosphere. SCWP targets areas that may harbor renegade electromagnetic fields and even disharmonious human activity. With minute scalar waves, it grounds abnormal currents, helping to manifest zero-point gravity.

Cold Laser

Most people, when hearing the term "medical laser," think about surgery. In fact, its use has revolutionized the surgeon's abilities. What we apply here at the Institute is a cold laser that does not bring mass light to a minute pinpoint but, in reverse, takes a pinpoint and spreads it out to a full spectrum. All lasers mimic the proton/photon function from the sun. When a cold laser (non-surgical) is applied over a certain region of the body, it figuratively slaps the system back into order. As a non-invasive tool, the recipient does not feel the subtle yet powerful process.

We are now several generations from the original technology used in the 20th century. As quantum physicists further delve into the principles that govern the multiple universes, they retrieve greater knowledge, expanding this technological field. Governments are reluctant to approve its use for more than cursory health concerns, although there is landmark evidence revealing that correctly applied lasers provide fruitful benefits for a wide variety of maladies.[297] More and more, you will see cold lasers applied when people seek to remedy ailments from as little as discomfort all the way to stage four disorders.

NuCalm

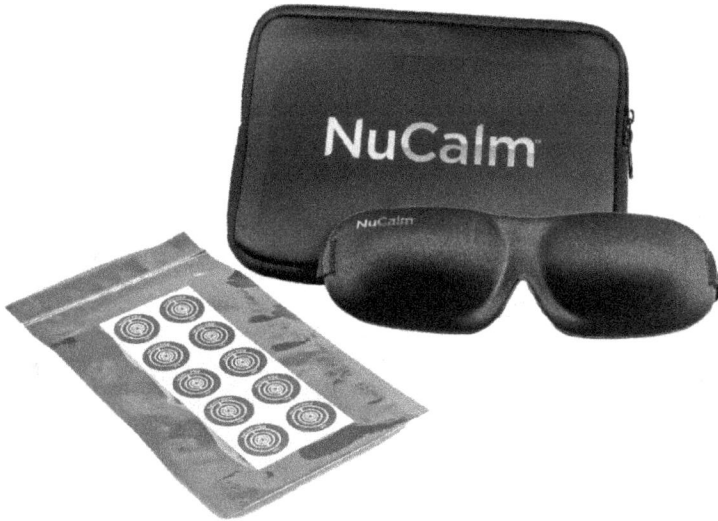

Source: https://store.nucalm.com/

This therapy is an advanced, non-invasive, drug-free solution designed to help you relax, restore, and achieve mental clarity. This cutting-edge therapy uses patented neuroscience technology to promote deep relaxation and reduce stress by guiding your brain into a state of balance and calm, also known as brainwave entrainment. Through the use of light and sound, NuCalm delivers a revolutionary approach to improving sleep, focus, and overall cognitive function.

NuCalm Therapy operates through a specially designed headset that delivers light and sound stimulation to help your brain reach a state of deep relaxation. The therapy is backed by over 35 years of research and involves a precise combination of frequencies that synchronize with your brainwaves. As your brain naturally aligns with these frequencies, stress and anxiety dissipate, allowing you to achieve mental calm and balance. NuCalm has been clinically proven[298] to lower stress, improve sleep quality, and enhance mental performance without the use of drugs or invasive techniques.

NuCalm is a comprehensive tool for mental recovery and performance enhancement. Whether you're dealing with chronic stress, anxiety, insomnia, or simply seeking better mental focus, NuCalm can help you achieve your goals.

A typical NuCalm session lasts about 20 to 30 minutes. You'll start by settling into a comfortable, quiet space where you can transition into a deeply relaxed state. As the session progresses, you'll experience a sensation of calm as your brainwaves synchronize with the gentle rhythms of the NuCalm system.

Tesla Plasma Frequency Machine:

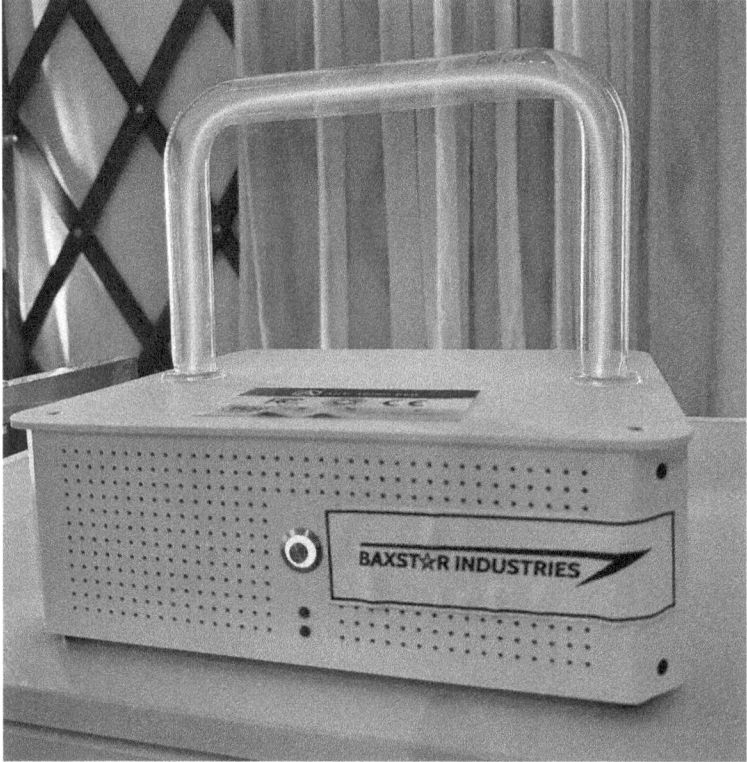

This advanced energy medicine device offers more than 500 programs and 4 million unique frequencies that Quantum Physics has discovered. The medicinal and therapeutic benefits of these currents, over the last century, have been validated. What makes this state-of-the-art technology is personalized protocols that address a plethora of concerns ranging from autism to mental illness, mold, arthritis, lime disease, many chronic diseases, and even cancer. Its engine is pulsed electromagnetic fields (PEMF). It also projects sound and light, which was spawned from the brilliant work of Nikola Tesla and other pioneers in this emerging medical field, like Nogier's, Royal Raymond Rife, and Hilda Clark, each of whom contributed science on frequencies that specifically targeted certain maladies. This plasma device is a compilation of tested and proven healing pulses gathered from multiple regions and cultures. My evaluation at the time of this writing is that this is the most advanced technology available today and can be easily utilized at home or in medical settings.

A New Frontier of Healing

We are just beginning to diagnose and treat using the frequency-based body. This field will only continue to grow. These non-invasive energy-based therapies render positive potential with no side effects.

This intricate blueprint of the invisible wiring that extends throughout the body affords a map to be utilized by modern electronic treatments.

One unique system that makes use of electrical information associated with the acupuncture points is the Motoyama AMI Machine.[299] Utilizing electrodes which attach to the terminal acupoints of the twelve main meridians, the AMI Machine is able to compare the electrical balance between the right and left sides of the body electrically unbalanced acupoints, as diagnosed by the AMI Machine, appear to reflect the presence of existing or impending disease in organ systems that are associated with those meridians.

This system, which is beginning to grow in popularity among doctors and dentists, is a device known as the Dermatron or Voll Machine[300]. The prototype of this system was developed by Dr. Reinhard Voll, a German physician. This technique is also known as EAV, or Electro-Acupuncture[301] according to Voll. Instead of solely monitoring the terminal acupoints of the meridians by remote computer measurement, as in the AMI system, the Voll device allows one to measure the electrical parameters of any acupuncture point in the body the Voll Machine is capable of going beyond the diagnosis of energetic imbalance levels in particular systems. It is frequently capable of finding the actual causes of the energetic dysfunction and potential help for the disorders. The manner in which the Voll Machine is able to carry out this type of analysis is a function of biological resonance the phenomenon of resonance is the principle behind the imaging systems of MRI and EMR scanning atoms and molecules have special resonant frequencies that will only be excited by energies of very precise vibratory characteristics it was postulated that homeopathic medicines contained an energy essence of the plant or other substance from which they were prepared. The energy essence of homeopathic medicine carries a type of subtle-energy signature of a particular frequency.

An electrotherapeutic approach to treating certain cancers was the focus of work by Dr. Bjorn Nordenstrom[302], the former head of Diagnostic Radiology at Stockholm's Karolinska Institute. Over the last several decades, Dr. Nordenstrom explored the use of specially applied electrical currents to treat cancer. In a limited number of patients, Dr. Nordenstrom was successful in producing complete remission from various types of this disease, metastatic to the lung.[303]

Nordenstrom utilized a number of mechanisms to explain why electrotherapy may be successful in destroying tumors. He discovered that white blood cells carry a negative electrical charge.[304] These tumor-fighting lymphocytes, he suggests, are drawn to the site of the cancer by the positive electrical charge of the platinum electrode in the center of the metastatic lesion. Therapeutically, a negative electrode is placed into normal tissue adjacent to the tumor. The resulting electrical field induces ionic tissue changes and buildup of acids in the local environment of the tumor, which are detrimental to the cancer cells.

Dr. Nordenstrom felt that bioelectrical circuits are part of an unexplored pulse circulatory system in the body. These natural electrical circuits switch on via injuries, infections, tumors, as well as the normal deconstruction and reconstruction of a balanced cellular system. Nordenstrom, like other bioenergetic researchers, agrees that disturbances in the bioelectrical network are involved in the development of cancer and other diseases.[305]

The Self-Care Movement Has Gone Electromagnetic

A pioneer in the science of bio-energy is Beverly Rubik[306], PhD, who earned her doctorate in biophysics from the University of California at Berkeley. She specializes in subtle energies for health and healing; she postulated in a paper published by the Foundation for Alternative and Integrative Medicine a case for what is needed in the further development of human bio-field measurement and other energetic instruments.[307]

She reviewed developments in three categories of bio-field measurement from humans: high-voltage electrophotography (the gas discharge visualization camera), electrodermal testing (EDT), and natural light emission (biophotons.) She called EDT the "more clinically useful" of the three methods, whereas the other two "are largely still tools for exploration in basic clinical research" with fewer applications.

Dr. Rubik's frustration is a seeming lack of interest from the scientific community to delve into this future medicine. Russians and Germans lead medical science in producing validated data highlighting the extraordinary multifaceted uses of subtle energy. "Modern Healthcare" generates economy from the chemical model.

When studying the origins of scientific excellence in energy medicine from the Eastern Bloc countries, there is a powerful emphasis on this advanced science in comparison to Western countries. Germany also has widely explored this future medicine with outstanding results. Ancients using geometry, geometric patterns, and nature's bountiful reserve of electrical stimuli consistently applied energy in healing.

Ben Franklin, America's key founder, hypothesized the powerful potential that electricity displays in the quest of the cause of physical disease.[308] We cannot allow language to dissuade us from moving forward wholeheartedly and embracing technologies that will liberate us from the shackles of chemically based paradigms.

In spite of the absence of English data, Dr. Rubik remains optimistic that "a large influx of funding for bio-field science" can move support for the existence of a human bio-field from the theoretical and experimental into the realm of everyday practical use. Recognize that there may be financial motivations discouraging scientists from exploring research that could reduce or eliminate the need for products produced by the so-called "health care" industry. Indeed, in other areas of medicine, an electromagnetic revolution is underway in the creation of hand-held devices or body-adorning technology for diagnostic use by healthcare consumers.

Mobile Cyber Health

While thousands of medical-related apps for smartphones have been produced to keep track of foods consumed and calories burned, only a few hundred contain sensors capable of making clinical measurements, such as blood glucose levels and blood pressure. Mobile Cyber Health (mHealth) involves medical technology on smartphones that can monitor vital signs and capture physiologic measurements, which can be of use to physicians and healthcare consumers alike.

Portable medical diagnostic devices containing artificial intelligence must be approved and regulated by the U.S. Food and Drug Administration if they are clinical-grade apps involving patient diagnostics. These would include apps enabling a healthcare professional to make a diagnosis using a medical image from a smartphone, an app that turns a smartphone into an ECG machine to detect abnormal heart rhythms, or an app with a blood glucose strip reader that functions as a glucose meter.

Unregulated apps that do not require FDA oversight are those that offer patient education and help consumers keep track of their health, mainly in the realms of fitness and nutrition. There are multitudes of up-and-coming technologies to track and aid in electromagnetic healthcare. One of these technologies would be an app that can test the nutritional viability

CHAPTER 14:

Your Frequency Vibrates Universal Energy

If you want to find the secrets of the universe, think in terms of energy, frequency, and vibration. - Nikola Tesla

For years, I have studied the emerging future science of quantum biology, recognizing that our failures in the healthcare field come, in large measure, from our inability to look deeply enough into what truly governs health and human existence.

A preoccupation with appearance and perception – as well as a limited imagination – have propelled humanity into a deep sense of insecurity. This has led us to disconnect from the totality of planetary life. Restrictive control has grown from this, as well as the need to categorize, compartmentalize, and isolate ourselves from the balanced rhythm that gives rise to all harmonious life.

Disorder and one of its step children, disease, has grown into the so-called 'norm.' Look at not only our lives, but the life of the planet. We and it have been affected by this disconnect. Oxygen and water are the two most important components for survival.

We are only now beginning comprehensive investigations into understanding the intricacies of these essential factors. Air/oxygen's prana has been revered since early man as the life force that maintains well-being.[311] Water directly collects energy from the sun at a greater level of frequency since it has less structure than solio-matter. This form of energy is essential to maintaining all life. Its invisible nano elements also collect ionic frequency at a pinnacle level, affording greater nourishment in all ways.[312]

In molecular science we purport that the larger the mass, the more energy it contains. While in fact, the less structure, the more energy abounds. Near nothingness contains an endless reservoir of constant frequency interactions from the connectedness linking us all together. This is why there is a limitless and eternally abundant amount of pulsation that can be tapped into when no matter or structure is holding it back.

As Dr. Joe Dispenza stated in his book *You Are the Placebo,* "Since the quantum field is an invisible field of information, it is frequency beyond space and time that all things material come from, and is made of consciousness and energy, whereas everything physical in the universe is unified within and connected to this field…you and I, along with all things in the multiple universes, are bonded by this field of intelligence… this is the systemic wisdom that's giving you life right now." [313]

In 1982, photographic research was conducted at UCLA exposing the connectivity with the external environment (universe) and our human bio-frequency fields. One of the most remarkable visuals appearing on the chromium film is when we are close to the ocean. There is a palpable connection between the movement of the waves and your personal frequency. The human body's electromagnetic field is negatively charged or ionized. When in close proximity to waves (tumbling water), which emit negative ions, increased electrical charges occur throughout our anatomy, expanding and enhancing our frequency fields. No wonder that a day at the beach feels so exhilarating and vitalizing. The same occurs between you and all-natural environments. Inversely, disharmonious and chaotic surroundings deplete our vital energy.

We all love a flowing brook, the freshness of outdoor vegetation, and the mountains. From our research at the Institute, as an example, we have dedicated extensive time, effort, and funds to the vegetation and natural ambiance of our campus, fostering a healing ecological setting.

Not only have we planted thousands of trees, but we have water features strategically placed along our nature trails and numerous pools. Inspirational art also dots the landscape. We used ancient energy geometry when erecting many of the structures and have built round dwellings as often as it seemed favorable. We had experts test the property as to what would be the best locations to nestle our residences and workplaces.

Additionally, we have placed pioneering scalar wave technology throughout the acreage to abolish the negative impact of WiFi and 5G. All of this is, in part, how our participants create biological and psychological balance, which accelerates the rebuilding of their immune systems. We discovered that living plants and a rarefied atmosphere create a richer field of negative ions to heighten and replenish our own energy field. When in such surroundings, our internal frequency becomes light in color and high in energy, sparkling and radiating out expansively from the body.

Add in nutrition and we have a key biological force and a clear example of how energetic totality works. Photons directly from the sun captured into your body by exposure, charges your system. Consuming uncooked plants that are drenched with these photons further enhances the electric pulsation of all your cells. Once the living vegetation has supplied its energetic nutritional properties it will then move to a secondary cycle, being composted, affording the soil the elements to recreate life. The process of decomposition generates proteins, vitamins, minerals, electromagnetic frequencies, and bacteria, nourishing plants as they grow, collecting more ionic energy from the Total. This is the heart of the cycle of life.

Procreation is our primary driving force as humans. This primal propulsion is the framework for all our thoughts, actions, and involvements throughout our existence. When this essential force is not nourished, we plunge further into despair. That is why connecting and mixing our energy fields with other humans and sharing a loving, supportive relationship enhances our strength, longevity, and healing power.

Psychologists have reported from extensive global studies that few people share happy and healthy partnerships. Deepening the schism is the technological age that has many engulfed in a cyber world most often directed by handheld technology. This continuous unnatural interaction robs us of precious time that historically has been spent on relationships including love, friendship, family, etc.

A perfect storm appears when we succumb to the unnatural and man-created fiascos of material disillusionment, corporate manipulation of our time, and the lethargy that these pseudo-luxuries encourage. It's important to remain dedicated to the true values that are born from your heart's epicenter. Our heart is the core driver of our positive interactions with the world around us.

Energy is information.

All energy medicine involves a variety of levels of light. This field of science indicates that the subtle light of consciousness contains the greatest healing potential, able to switch on and off the biochemical and biophysical processes in our bodies at a cellular level.

During the 20th century, all major life processes were thought to be chemical in nature[314]; in the 21st century, these life processes are being redefined as electromagnetic in nature[315]. For example, energy medicine is less expensive, safer, and a non-intrusive alternative to chemical medicine. It traces its origins to the traditional systems of Homeopathy, Ayurveda, and Chinese medicine, whose essence rely on the idea of bio-fields that radiate bio-energy (qi, prana, vital force) that can be enhanced.

As the noted Chief Seattle from the Duwamish tribe once stated, "the earth does not belong to man; man belongs to the earth[316], and it is for us to be sensible, from our heart outward, to all other life on this planet." He and other Indigenous people saw life force and energy in all of nature. They respectfully voiced gratitude for being part of the comprehensive ecology of Earth.

Modern people seem to have lost this sense of oneness with everything and pride themselves on egocentric individualism. We have even fooled ourselves into believing that we should kill for survival without any consequences. The consumption of animals and their milk is one bizarre example of how estranged we are from the reality of planetary life force and the interconnections of all life forms. By relinquishing this horrific practice, we can show the required respect and allow the planet to begin mending.

Quantum biology has led us to see that all reality is self-created and expressed via internal imagination and creation and external reflection of that realized intention. We are each universes connected to the limitless universes that flow in one positive direction. To master our purpose, we must learn how to interact with respect and patience not only with all other people but with each and every life, environment, ecosystem, and event. Navigating gracefully is our birthright and can be easily achieved once you realize that ideas express your current reality but can vary and change within a split second. For this reason, a humbling, heart-felt relationship with others should be pursued since all of us are in constant flux. Our unity with life will empower our bodies and minds to maintain utmost health, happiness, and healing!

We welcome you to participate in the new world of quantum biology, which will revolutionize the future of disease eradication and optimal health maintenance.

We all stand at a precipice relating to tomorrow. Abundant magnificence is always accessible when self-imposed ideals, norms, and social mores are shattered. Remaining entrapped in a molded history and cultural dogma, our true self is not in play, which prevents enriching progress from occurring. For this reason, disassembling the grips of preconceived notions is the first step in chartering stagnation which is required for powerful health. From the exploration that you have undertaken when ingesting the words assembled in this offering, I hope it ignites a plethora of possibilities that you are committed to acquiring. Whether it is building personal trust or the next game-changing technology, you are the "Michaelangelo" of your destiny.

You are a gathering of billions of moving parts, thoughts, actions, emotions, spiritual aspirations, etc. Unifying the orchestra of these invaluable components are what manifests a thriving life. Fueling your pursuit to a purposeful future requires formidable passion. Being "All In" before you begin is a prerequisite to each and every success, be it biological, psychological, or spiritual. All too often, rituals and rhetoric cloud the pathway and create a false sense of enlightenment. Humanity has institutionalized, incorporated, and prostituted every potential legitimate avenue to consciousness.

Always being taught to aspire to do too little and conform by embracing and practicing others' theories has squashed the joy of authentic expression. We all routinely surrender our progress to mediocre re-runs of repetitive processes. Ironically, those who are the best at mimicking are revered as the wise, whereas often, the seemingly strange, awkward, and wacky one out in left field is actually the one tuned in to the abundance channel. Everything good is new and untarnished, and inspiration is generated by passion. Our social mores and hierarchical institutions surely limit and prevent innovation and unbridled achievement.

When seeing everything as particles of energy that move from invisible to the actual structure, you will enable the mind to drop the pretense and create masterpieces. Every thing, thought, blade of grass, rocket ship, flower bud, and steel bridge are unified frequencies that organically establish form and function. Your ability to internalize this truth will empower you with the enthusiasm to manufacture all affirmative thoughts into reality.

One of the architects of Quantum Theory, Niels Bohr stated that "reality is none of his business."[317] He was just exposing the mix-up of what is available to employ when you create reality.

Whether you know it or not, you have been doing this throughout your entire life. Seemingly, we take this profound occurrence in a less than serious way. Imagine what will happen when you exercise your ability to create empowering purposeful events. Solutions rather than problems, success rather than failure, and healing rather than disorder. This is all inherent as a birthright for every person on earth, few possess the graceful gratitude to utilize this profound endowment.

Recently, I met with a woman whom I had the privilege of guiding two decades ago and was amazed at how markedly transformed she was in comparison to when she and her husband first sat at my desk. At that time, it was difficult for her to focus or even sit up. Clearly, she was suffering from severe cognitive issues, yet, I never suspected it could be a tumor weighing more than the brain itself.

Her prognosis was grim, and even the 'renowned attending physicians' expressed that there was no hope and that she should thus go home and prepare for her imminent demise.

Although I have spent decades working with seriously conscious and seriously ill people, seldom have I observed the combination. She displayed how affirmative imagination, utter commitment to a healing lifestyle, and spiritual application can conquer such a malady. These enigmas are titled spontaneous remission, or a miracle, rather than the manifestation of desired reality.

Today, all of humanity stands at a threshold that fosters the return to majestic empowerment. Courage must be rendered to leave behind the institutionalized, limiting society and cultures that were poorly erected. All of our energy seems to have been drained from propping up a false narrative that we call life. It is this very act that has crushed and diminished us into a state of subservience. How freeing it is to wholeheartedly leave behind an entrapped existence and internalize the vast potential of imagined clarity.

Quantum Humans are the pinnacle members of our species who will guide us toward the vista representing infinite competence. Self-motivation, combined with potent skills, manifests positive results without fail. Concrete examples of this are sprinkled throughout human history. Unfortunately, most perceive this as an ideal that is just out of their reach. Now is the time to skillfully build an internal well of plentiful possibilities that can flow freely from an unbridled mind.

Steps to Quantum Realization

New frontiers also require a methodical process and committed organization. Your first step into the freedom of manifesting an abundant life requires baby steps. Think deeply and thoroughly about what is preventing you from embracing a joyous existence. It is this obstacle that has to be sanded away and formed into a sculpture of desired reality. We should never attempt to discard the particles that block us, but more so to take them and reformulate positive results out of the same energy.

As an example, if your greatest nemesis preventing happiness is your inability to move and exercise, you begin by committing to short brisk walks every day. Within reason as time passes, you can add more vigor and time to the practice. Next, you can integrate resistance exercise and stretching. All of this results in a psychological and biological change that is measurable and encouraging. With the passage of time, you will be residing in a functional body that is capable of achieving whatever your imagination wishes it to do. After practicing simple tasks of creation, you will be inspired to leap forward and strive for more significant challenges.

Visualization, in and of itself, may be the initial pursuit, yet it is massaging the dream into a viable accomplishment that matters. We now possess science revealing that light and sound move through thick walls. Why then is it so hard to create the cure for a disease or actualize a goal? As pieces of puzzles in disarray, we are impotent until we affix ourselves into the empty spaces and dimensions of a unified puzzle. One step and then the next will reveal the entire picture that is ultimately your desire.

Fearlessness is not always provoked by instinct but is most often available by believing in new possibilities and acknowledging previous success. People appearing as profits are no more than those mining their human reserves. Progress is made by affixing affirmative experience to affirmative experience. This new roadway will guide you into heightened acquisitions of fulfilling scenarios. Systematically, your basket will fill with accomplishments with universal roots in the scheme of existence. Unleashing your lesser self to become a generous philanthropist of love and harmony assures you a deserved seat at the human table. Our banquet is to be distributed among all others so the nourishment strengthens our species and pole vaults us into the world that is meant to be. This is not utopic but a successful pursuit that allows for peaceful and prosperous circumstances to prevail. We do not have to believe discord is part of our condition. Why accept the burden of history as the inevitable future?

As a child, you were able to have conversations with imaginary friends, turn lemons into sweetness, and conveniently forget that you cannot fly. For this reason, it is for you to rekindle the spirited passion that results in euphoric contemplation. No pain, no gain is the outdated mode of a broken culture.

Today's quantum human has shed the armor of protection and adorned their spirit with bright illuminous energy. This energy can burn through steel, respect and honor a butterfly, and establish global oneness. We have all had glimpses of greatness in the past, yet have fallen short of residing in its glory permanently.

Negative events should be considered oddities rather than the "normal" state of affairs. What is normal, then? It is what you believe it is. What is real is what you create. What is viable for you and all others? We are eternally bonded, and for this reason, as we crawl out of the ditches that we have dug, we will raise everyone along with us. With feet securely affixed to the ground we then can ascend to the higher self that we have missed for most of our lives.

CHAPTER 15:

Quantum Living

For the first time in history, today's human is immersed in a reality that so rapidly unfolds, morphs, and changes that it creates a sense of insecurity and confusion. As you have read in the chapters before this, we are a gathering of frequencies that form our biology, mentality, emotions, and interaction with others and all life.

At this time, you have to rethink your approach to enhancing your existence so that well-being, productivity, and contribution are achieved with the highest level of integrity. This requires diligence that most likely supersedes the casual commitments you might have made in the past that have achieved some level of success. Your ability to personify the 21st-century human is essential at a time when the entire human race is challenged to remain in our natural evolutionary rhythm.

Everything that you thought making you special is now in a battle that can only be won by a person who appreciates and respects the soulful depth of connectivity to the greater multiple universes. We are already becoming dependent upon electronic consciousness[318], which includes memory, knowledge, and even wisdom. This inherently will lead an on-seasoned person into a robotic state. The opportunity for the powers to disassemble you and all others has never been greater. As we know, robots can be programmed to do whatever is desired[319]; they do not require love, empathy, compassion, or even traditional food. Hybrid versions of this currently exist. Yet, with the massively growing competence of artificial intelligence, I anticipate that this takeover of the human spirit is imminent.

Maintaining your humanity is achievable with the daily practices and systems that I have established over the last half-century. We must maintain our connection with the natural world and always be unified with the umbilical cord of the universe. Fundamental to your liberation from this estranged period is your willingness to commit yourself to strong, clear, and honest values.

Seven requirements to achieve quantum human status
One

- Discovering, embracing, and establishing your life's purpose.
- Primarily extending all of your energy and time in pursuing this passion.
- Developing confidence and proficiency in your contribution.

What is most often overlooked in parenting, education, and work is that people feel imposed upon when they are fulfilling someone else's needs and/or agenda.

Purposeful, passionate life missions not only fulfill you, but also contribute to helping others and improving the overall human condition.

Two

- Fueling your body and consciousness with nutrition and mental focus.
- Establishing daily disciplines that do not restrict your progress but give it a basis to grow.
- Creating a life balance between passionate /contribution, intimate/ personal relationships and renewal/regeneration.

Three

- Upload pertinent knowledge and experiential enhancement.
- Leave your comfort zone to abolish fear.
- Pursue, challenge and interrelate with people who may not agree.

Four

- Create home and work environments that are suited to free your expression
- Surround yourself with art, music, literature, and performances that enrich you.
- Always be willing to change when feeling trapped in your current environment/surroundings.

Five

- Allow yourself to be comfortable with rest and relaxation as much as success.
- Make your heart the emperor of your life.
- Embrace love as power and anger/manipulation as the enemy

Six

- Authentic and honest relationships should be your benchmark.
- Your every expression should be pure, candid, and spontaneous.
- Recognize freedom as your North Star.

Seven

- Prepare to live beyond a century.
- Develop a history and legacy that enriches future generations
- Gratitude should always be your go to place in times of trouble and accomplishment.

Achieving quantum humanity

The twenty-one clear rules mentioned above will enrich and empower you to live at the necessary quantum level to thrive at this time in history. Granted, many of these choices are not conventional and/or familiar; they have been practiced by the greatest leaders and visionaries throughout history. As Norman Vincent Peale[320], the pioneering motivational provocateur stated, "Without a humble but reasonable confidence in your own powers you cannot be successful or happy." [321]

To lose one's self at this moment, is easier than it has ever been. Ironically, at the same time, it is easier to live your true created reality than it ever has been before. The difference between a core commitment to BEING versus a need to be part of something is the disparity that will either ignite your persona or cause you to completely eliminate yourself. All of us should aspire to a species-wide engagement of self-realization. This will then shield us from the engaging negativity that those living in a lesser state of awareness impose. There is an opportunity for us to burgeon into beings of light that have the foremost objective of bringing peace and balance.

Examples of quantum life

- Start each day by listing three significant goals either mentally or in writing with a sincere objective to achieve them.
- Ideally, consume only pure/ distilled water and/or raw, fresh, non-sugary juices along with supplementation in place of breakfast.
- Schedule and achieve an exercise/movement program daily.

A: Resistant exercise three days a week for a minimum of 90 minutes.

B: Aerobic exercise for 35 minutes - a minimum of 5 days per week.

C: Stretching/ yoga/Pilates/swimming - every day for 15 minutes.

Examples of quantum life, continued

- Before and/or during important decision-making, breathe deeply and spend 15-30 seconds asking your soul which decision is best.

- When sitting in contribution/work, always stand and walk for one minute, every 20 minutes.

- Know your strengths and find people who are passionate enough to help you in your pursuits or who are themselves also passionate in those areas.

- Ideally take one hour break for lunch time and make this the largest meal of the day. By pursuing this important nutritional goal, you will fuel the body at a time it is most able to digest and absorb nutrients. The 11:30 am - 1:30 pm window is the best for this to occur. Your food choices must be organic, fresh, and, in great part, raw. Plant-based food is essential because any other fare detracts from biological, psychological, and universal functions.

- In the afternoons, when the sun is abundant and photonic energy is significantly available, it is good to work/contribute in a space with poly glass rather than regular glass so the sun rays enter the room and/or to simply move outdoors. If neither is available, take a break in the midafternoon, no matter where you live on the planet, and spend 15 minutes a day outside taking a walk.

- Always adorn your body with organic undergarments and ideally organic clothing. At the very least, only purchase 100% natural fiber garments so that your body can breathe and when exposed to the elements, the man made chemically created garments will not be pouring estrogenic endocrine disruptors into your system.

- As often as possible, walk with bare feet on the earth and use cloth or natural soles so that you connect and ground your body.

- When consuming dinner it must be organic, plant-based, fresh and in great part, uncooked. Portions should be small as the body's circadian rhythm, and digestive function slow down in the evening and night, making it harder to utilize nutrients as effectively as earlier in the day. Additionally, you do not want to eat and then retire. There should always be 3-4 hours between eating and sleeping.

- Providing you do not suffer from an eating disorder or emaciation from medical treatments, part of your weekly schedule should be a 24-hour fast. This should include juices from green leafy vegetables, excluding any high-sugar varieties like carrots, beets, or fruits. In addition, you can drink clean distilled water that can include fresh lemon juice and/or coconut water.

- When entertaining yourself in the evening, make sure it does not involve computers, cell phones, or computer screens/TVs, which emit brain and immune-altering electronic waves. These unfamiliar frequencies confuse the body's organs and nervous system which is governed by the brain. Resultingly, sleep will not be of high quality, and immunity will not be as strong. There are EMF devices that help to protect you from the renegade frequencies that technology brings.

- Artificial light that pours from our cities, towns, and villages skews our brain's balance and connectivity to the stars and abundant skies that guided our ancestors for millennia. Visiting remote regions of the planet and re-engaging with the womb of nature will recalibrate your neurological system and re-regulate your brain so that mental clarity and sleep patterns can be reinstituted.

- Before retiring, spend 5 minutes in a mindfulness practice and 5 minutes writing down in a special notebook with the title of your choice, similar to the "ME BOOK." You should note down the seven things that you liked most about yourself that day. This should take no more than a few words and a few minutes. This simple yet profound daily practice accrues forty-nine affirmative thoughts a week, approximately two hundred a month, and at the end of the year, more than two thousand. This is a proven technique that, when habitually employed, recalibrates mindset, brain pathways, and attitude. As important as it is to eat living food to energize a living body, positive thought nurtures a healthy and productive mind and soul.

- Make sure you are in a cool, fully darkened room with comfortable and healthy organic bedding. Plan to sleep uninterrupted at least 8 hours nightly. If you find this difficult to begin with before training, you may want to employ advanced technologies like NuCalm and BrainTap. This is science-based energy medicine that has broken through even the worst cases of insomnia. Recognize that sleep and longevity are as many healing partners as proper nutrition and exercise are for a long life.

- When contribution and work are your passion, it is easy not to break away and make time to be at total rest and peace. Quantum humanity requires periodic breaks that change the cyclical patterns that can inherently trap you and limit your progress. By removing yourself from routines, you force helicopter vision and widen your vista so that when you re-engage, limitlessness sparks a refreshing, enthusiastic future aspiration.

Fuel stops for healing well being and consciousness

More than a century ago, science began to acquire knowledge about treatments, therapies, lifestyle, engagement, and the ability to charge and recharge ourselves. When understanding our purpose is the most basic way, it is like a pristine battery (body, mind, soul) that needs energy to keep functioning. Contemporary life is a minefield of energy detraction and massive energy output. For this reason, there are specific proven methods that will continually renew us, affording exceptional frequency to thrive so we can contribute at the highest level. Long, healthy, and happy lives are achieved when we plug into these gifts.

Listed below are practices that are rated from 1-10 with 10 being the maximum to increase lifeforce and longevity.

Forrest/Nature bathing a minimum of 3 days per week for 1 hour. This is commonly practiced in Japan, and you achieve an increase of energy via the sun and cosmic rays that build immune and neuron cell strength. **(7)**

Swimming - bathing in oceans, rivers, streams, ponds, and lakes. This practice, in immersing in the earth's bloodstream, vitalizes and recharges your frequency fields that are circulating in your vascular plasma. Saltwater charges a bit higher at **(8)**. Whereas small bodies of fresh water **(6)**, **(7)** active fresh waters, rivers, and large lakes. Depending on your location and climate, you can swim or bathe in natural settings whenever possible. Water at temperatures between 35 and 45 super invigorates the nervous system and lymph glands and provokes increased immune cell activity. Spending 3 minutes submerged in this ice water is a **(9)**

Nudity/Clothing - Sunbathing year around in early morning and late day charges the body's battery fully. When temperatures are too cold to be nude or near nude, adorn your body with organic/natural fiber clothing where there may be a 15-25% reduction in photon intake. Depending upon the garments, **(8/9)**.

Scandinavian saunas, far and near-infrared saunas, steam baths, and whirlpool tubs. Bodies of evidence from the scientific community reveal the detoxification and cell-enhancing benefits of these traditional and accessible therapies. Once considered a luxury, today's Quantum Human should add these enhancement treatments to their daily life. Scandinavian (**6**) Far infrared (**8**) Steam baths (**6**) Whirlpools (**5**).

Walking and climbing These two natural and desirable aerobic endeavors have surfaced as universally the most beneficial for overall health. Walking briskly for as little as 10 minutes can add years to your life and clarity to your mind. Climbing stairs, trees, or mountains combines body-strengthening exercises with aerobics and can benefit you on several levels. There is a psycho/bio enhancement from natural movements stemming from evolutionary development. Neurocise is Hippocrates' developed fitness program that is foremost incomprehensibly unifying anatomy, psychology and spirituality. Walking hopefully for a minimum of 20 minutes 5 days per week, is a solid (**6**). Climbing for a minimum of 3 days per week even if it is a long staircase affords a (**7**). Neurocise (**10**).

Dancing/Sports These expressive movements connect the heart and soul, infusing inherent energy with bodily systems. Depending upon the duration and commitment, (**6-9**).

Art - Music, Visual Arts, Theater, Spoken word, Motion Pictures. These passionate pursuits that you either participate in or observe, unlock your spirit and spark imaginative thoughts that engage your engine of passion. This provokes (**5-9**), depending upon the level of participation you have either as the artist or audience.

Personal Relationships. Be it love, family, or close friends, this area of endeavor has become a focus for those desiring a long life. Healthy relationships enhance your lifespan with individual or group support, renders a sense of security that allows your persona to soar and your anatomy to function in a relaxed and symbiotic way (**5-7**).

Passionate Work. As rare as this is, with only 23% of the global public stating that they "love what they do," to make a living it is as important if not more important than most other areas of our lives. Since the average person spends more than 40 hours per week at work, and many hours more resting and recovering to go back to work, finding what you love where it does not appear or feel like work can supercharge your existence (**8-10**).

Organic food-based supplementation. The emerging science of nutriceuticals has given us a concise roadmap to enhancing overall health via nourishing systems of the body through life filled nutrients. All supplements must be unheated, allowing the lifeforce locked into the cells of the organic plants to interact and interrelate with your body's cells. Think of these desirable supplements as condensed packages of food which further supports the proper functions of your anatomy and psychology (**7-10**).

Body work/Touch therapy/Reiki When a balanced and well-seasoned body worker or touch therapy reiki expert engages with you, their confident and focused energy literally enhances your body's electromagnetic field. Psychoneuroimmunology is a perfect description of what occurs when you are undergoing massage/touch treatments. It not only calms the mind but activates the nervous system, which enters every organ of the body and sparks the immune system to do its job (**7-9**).

Energy Medicine/ Magnetic—Sound, Light, Cold Laser. This growing science-based future medicine permits noninvasive treatments to permeate your bodily systems, resulting in affirmative outcomes to balance organs, strengthen glands, clarify the neurological system, and unify the totality of the body. Everything from pain to emotional upheaval to immune disorder can be successfully helped without the implementation of chemistry since you are an electromagnetic body (**8-10**).

Mindfulness Practices Tapping, Breathing, Body Scan, Tai Chi, Yoga, Meditation etc. Each of these techniques can take away the noise, settle the mind, and allow concise focus on your desired goal. Current research shows that this enhances the total body balance required to maintain functional systems and superior health. One example is within 5 minutes of devoted application to one of these practices, there can be up to 40 percent more immune cell activity (**6-9**).

Journaling and writing. Although people need psychotherapy to heal lifetime wounds, self-help methods like journaling achieve similar results. Purging the mind, which affects the body, is as important as any healing technique, and Quantum humans will increasingly embrace this practice. (**5-7**).

Sound therapy. Moving water, raindrops, birds, wind, nature, children's laughter – all of this delightful audio experience opens our hearts and minds and triggers our connectivity to the greater whole. By once again rooting ourselves in the origins of existence, we become significantly stable and confident in our purpose. For this reason, it charges the mind/body (**5-7**).

Life Enhancement Wisdom. Be it a motivational speaker, a spiritual practice, or an inspirational gathering/workshop, your universal connection to all other people and the universal desire we have to love and be loved can be greatly enriched by participating in mind-provoking and spirit sparking events (**5-7**).

Resistant exercise. Hatha Yoga, Endurance Exercise, Weight Lifting - Each develops stronger, larger, and more elastic muscular bodies. This essential practice should be conducted throughout life and not only builds stronger bones and organ systems, but also strengthens mentality, expands longevity and protects memory, cardiovascular health, as well as sexuality (**6-8**).

Extreme pursuits to abolish fear by placing yourself in a safe yet frightening act. (Skydiving, firewalking, bungee jumping, scuba diving, public speaking, etc.), can successfully demolish self-constructed barriers of limitation. As an example, the fear of flying has often been corrected by interacting with a flight simulator until you reprogram the brain, freeing it from the fear.

> **Mirror exercises.** Where you look directly into your own eyes and have a conversation with yourself about "problems, concerns, reluctance, self-sabotage etc., until you reach a point of agreement on why these obstacles exist is an extremely effective way to expand your potentiality and humanity.

Crushing lack of confidence and self-expression by devaluing their own significance is a harsh and cruel reality for many. As boiling water in a kettle finally speaks out by whistling, you have to acquire self-respect, which participates in confidence that inevitably creates a release of oppressive and unresolved emotional baggage. Speak the words that you are internalizing in the presence of others. Practice this until it becomes second nature for you to do this naturally and organically as life progresses. Be principled with pillars of unshakable commitment to your core belief representing your whole self.

Primal personalities have reigned until our now quantum humanity begins to bloom. In this time of history, our predesignated roles within the masculine and feminine mindset must be rethought. The feeble and dainty image of the feminine largely developed due to the disrespect that we have shown for women. Previously, women had to "out man" men to gain respect and so-called success. Quantum humans will embrace the polarity of strength and sensitivity, releasing themselves to free expression. We must also honor and respect biological differences between males and females and the need for most of us to be interdependent upon one another. Half a circle cannot roll gently through life. When combined with the other half, this mobility comes with ease, grace, sophistication, and power. Your process of balancing your left and right brain and your feminine and masculine self requires repetitive actions that define you to self and others. Like a great actor who memorizes their script confidently and fluidly articulates the self-realized personality that they have become.

Traditional psychology has categorically worked from the premise of corrective measures applied to your current life. Quantum science and humans acknowledge and effectively work in understanding that we are part of a perpetual and continual flow of energy that has emerged from eons of nothingness moving forward into a state of allness. We are a compilation of everything that has ever been, everything that is, and everything that will be. Both ancestral human and cosmic traits have, in great part, contributed to who you currently BELIEVE YOU ARE. Breaking this pattern is not only in great part psychological but more so spiritual and cosmic. All of this has to be taken into account when a permanent shift to a more affirmative you is the desired goal. This can be accomplished with psychedelic and quantum psych therapies. One must be cautious that it is not utilized as escapism but truly employed to achieve selfism.

Below is a basic example of what your day can look like once you are committed to raising your frequency. Leave behind the ideas of self-improvement, micronutrients, and disciplines to become spiritual. We are one that organically will afford you an increase in inner strength, physical well-being, emotional balance, and enhanced consciousness by following simple steps.

Quantum Day

Awaken: Touch your head, heart, and body gently as you observe your surroundings and melt into the environmental ambiance. Either move directly into sunlight or in the dark hours, employ full spectrum light in your home/environment.

Plan: Sit for 3-5 minutes, inhale deeply. Visualize what will fulfill you this day by defining your focus and use it to bring a sense of direction to the day ahead.

Organizational Clarity: Put in place any objects and make your bed as ancient feng shui teaches us, that an orderly dwelling brings a powerful persona.

Hydrate: Consume pure distilled water and/or mix it with fresh organic plant green juice. This is when we need to consume the most liquid since our bodies inherently dehydrate during rest and sleep. Fluid consumption also helps us evacuate the accumulated debris collected during the night.

Sparktrition: Morning is best to take high-frequency raw plant-based plantceuticals so that your cells are enriched by the electron frequencies that they ignite. Today's sophisticated genetic nutritional tests can expose what you need the most and those that you may ingest to heighten biological and consciousness activity. Phytonutrition that is unprocessed and filled with the photons from the sun via the photosynthesis process will always contain the highest proteins, minerals, and essential fatty acids. Additionally, they contain Hormones, Oxygen, Phytochemicals, and Enzymes. This is the era of HOPE in quantum nutrition.

Food: Ideally, you should not consume solid food until 11:30 a.m. This way, you harbor the energy that would normally go to digestion and elimination for physical, emotional, and consciousness exploration. If you are consuming fare, it must be organic, unprocessed, uncooked plants like seeds, nuts, grains, and beans, all in their germinated form.

Movement/Exercise/Fun: Daily stretching, aerobics, and every other day resistance exercise for 30 mins and 90 minutes need to be routine and correctly conducted. Modern humans require the same level of stamina harvested from exertion that previous generations had throughout human history. Circulatory blood and neurology activate glandular and organ systems needed to maintain their functioning, which expels exemplary biochemistry fueling body/mind balance. Maintaining youth, heart, brain, and libido capacity and expressing sexuality all depend upon a fit, flexible, and durable physique.

Hot/Cold: Immediately following vigorous exercise, spend a minimum of 20 minutes in, ideally, an infrared sauna or a minimally Scandinavian type. If available, cold plunge or cryotherapy (dry cold) for a maximum of 3 minutes builds on the benefits that exercise affords. These well-researched and scientifically established techniques expand lifespan, increase immune system cells and their function, as well as make you feel more relaxed after their detoxifying and neurologically stimulating effects. (Steam baths and/or Whirlpool tubs bring benefits, but to a lesser degree).

Mindfulness Chores: Clean up the kitchen area so that clutter is removed from your mind and work area. Create a habitual routine that comes naturally and effortlessly. CLEAR MIND CLEAR ABODE brings crystal clarity.

Mindful Work or Activity: Passionate pursuits are the only endeavors that conscious quantum people should pursue. It is simple to understand that those times that you spend in either work or activities that fulfill and enrich you are the most productive and rewarding. Old paradigms in positions led us to believe that working appropriately was difficult and, at times, even painful. This is the basis of why the old economy collapsed and why people's emotional, spiritual, and biological selves have been injured. IT IS NOT NO PAIN, NO GAIN, BUT CONVERSELY, ANY PAIN, NO GAIN. You must find purposeful employment that utilizes your contribution and energies so it results in personal and planetary rewards. No longer can we live in discord that participates in disharmony, in self, in family, in community, humanity, and planetary. We must eradicate the statistic that 80% of the global workforce is not congruent with what they do to "make a living." Your leisure, community, and athletic activities have to harmonize with your heart and soul. Otherwise, your lifeforce will be drained by the very thing that is supposed to afford you rest and renewal.

Evening Dining: When consuming more than one meal per day, your second or third meal will most likely be in the evening. Our bodies have evolved to need little or no food before 11:30 a.m. Then, the largest meal was consumed before 1:30 p.m. Late in the afternoon or early evening, a small portion dining was common. As you consciously grow, food is no longer your foremost fuel. So, as time passes, it is best to eat little or nothing in the early evening before sleeping.

Food such as raw salads, avocados, nut and seed preparations, plant-soups, and/or raw, low or no sugar juices are the essence of nutrition that the high frequency body requires.

Relaxation - PreSleep: Music, literature, family, and communal activities including games and walks in nature are all empowering activities that disconnect you from the electronic AI networks and help you reconnect with your human power and perceptual abilities, allowing you to expand well beyond your previously imagined limitations.

Building Self-Realization: The heart of a happy and productive life is drawn from the deepest gifts and greatest aspirations that you harbor. Our global society has disregarded this, unlike the ancient cultures of the East and West. Our drive to achieve material gain has squashed the desire to fulfill your purpose. Loving parents do not have the tools to lead you in the direction of self-realization, no less confused and broken souls that have given birth and do not even have the slightest idea of how to nurture their offspring. Generational inheritance is much broader than the material left behind but is actually spiritually genetic, where unresolved problems from your ancestors are part of your upbringing. Remarkably you have the ability to flush away all the dimensions that block you from thriving as a fully enlightened being.

Imagery is a tool that the most progressive minds in advance thinking apply to support the healing of those who feel themselves entrapped in their own current reality. You must be brave enough to create the ideal, acting consistently so you are not dissatisfied with your current thoughts and actions. We deflect our precious time by idealizing others rather than anointing ourselves as the greatest teachers, leaders, and humanitarians that have ever lived. **You are remarkably gifted, now it is time for you to express that in each and every action.**

Through this process, you will express the core values that allow you to liberate yourself from the perpetual patterns of brokenness. By embracing these simple methods, you can emerge and become soulfully content and inspirationally enriched to grow, give, and share. You are magnificent, awaiting a time to perform at your highest level of purity.

- Negativity reins and is used to market, suppress, silence, sell to, motivate, and frighten you. Quantum humans will estrange themselves from these deceptive practices and search out and live in and with affirmative people and environments. This includes family, work, socialization, and entertainment.

- Life is like a canoe trip. As you first enter the river, it is calm and gentle; as you row forward, you may hit rapids and, at times, even waterfalls. These experiences are inevitable and can create negative moments, yet they do not have to be incorporated permanently into yourself. All of this obviously affects you, yet it does not have to change you at your core. Learning to filter all experiences and develop affirmative thoughts about them will build your confidence, character stamina, and persona.

- One never reaches an optimum place of knowledge, consciousness, and wisdom, so it is important for you to pursue new experiences, learning, and esoteric exploration. Most people relish the past because they cannot see themselves in the future without the fuel of exciting endeavors moving forward. When one continues on an enriching path, the path leads us to a longer, more fulfilling life.

- Our society has molded us to be listeners from external sources. Meanwhile, the voice generated by your inner soul is the guiding light that will empower you to become a self-realized human. This voice cannot be manufactured through your mind's memories and habits. Its resonance is a clear and powerful emotion. Differentiate it from your persistent patterns of thought-creating action.

- Forgiveness is the antidote for regrets. You may feel that you are pursuing a failing challenge rather than enhancing your understanding from a new experience. Forgive yourself and remember that we are creatures in the process of becoming whole. Not whole in the process of unraveling.

- When feeling abused, recognize that the abuser is most often discombobulated mentally, emotionally, and spiritually. For this reason, do not internalize the punishment bestowed upon you as your own fault. Reality prevails that you, in this victim role, are able and capable of enduring the assault. So, find a way to grow beyond the pain and become a disciple of the goodness of man.

- Consciousness is divided into sub and current; sub is developed by experiences that create cyclical patterns that etch limitations into your psyche. Between conception and six and a half years old, most of the subconscious is created. So-called consciousness is about 5% that is easy to adjust via imagination, inspiration and exploration. This is where we can fill our heads up with knowledge that does not do a bit of good until we break the underlying habits of repeating thoughts, actions, and spiritual endeavors.

- Remain awake in congruence with your surrounding environment and chosen path. You are constantly connected to universal wisdom that will clearly guide you in the right direction. Most people lack the receptivity to embrace this invisible yet powerful force, so for that reason, their lower consciousness draws them back into the place of so-called "safety" preventing them from growth, fulfillment, and spiritual enhancement.

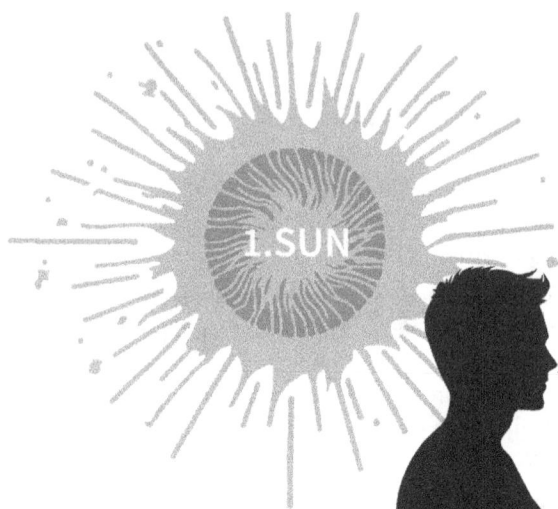

1. SUN

2. PHOTONS

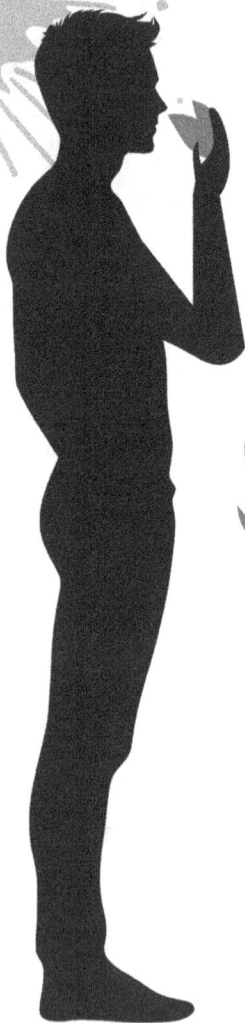

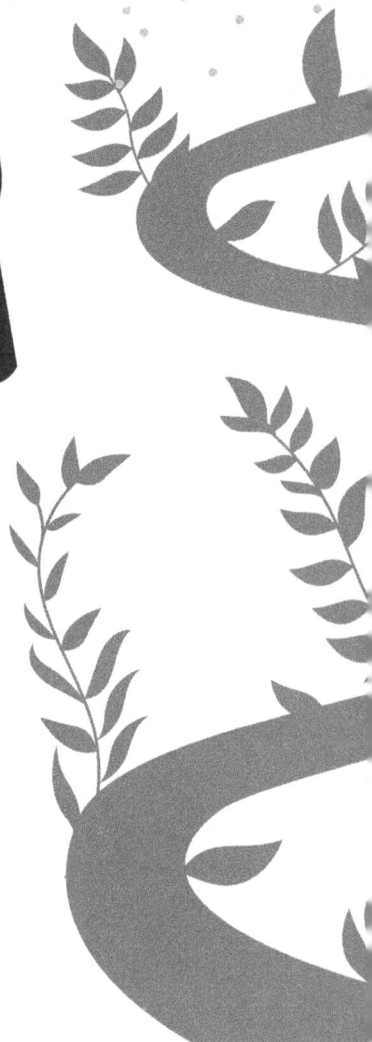

4. GREEN PLANT CONSUMPTION

3.PHOTOSYNTHESIS

5. CELLULAR ENERGY (FREQUENCY)

APPENDIX ONE:

Science Studies Relevant to Quantum Human Biology

"Non-local correlations between separated neural networks." Pizzi R. Et al. *Quantum Information and Computation II*, edited by Eric Donkor, Et al. Proceedings of SPIE. 2004.

In exploring quantum models for brain activity, five scientists at the University of Milan in Italy, did an experiment in which "two separated and completely shielded basins" were used containing "two parts of a common human DNA neuronal culture," monitored by an EEG machine. When one culture was stimulated by a laser beam, the other shielded culture displayed the same effects as the neurons exposed to the light, indicating a 'non-local' connection that persisted for the once joined neural cells. The research team was baffled by the 'cross-talk' effect, calling it "not explainable by classical models."

"New Nonlocal Biological Effect: A Preliminary Research." Hu H. Wu M. *NeuroQuantology*. 2012 September.

Biophysics scientists exposed Poland Spring water to one minute of 1500 Watts of microwaves, and then separated the water into two parts. Into half of the water, five tablets of Primatene, an over-the-counter medication for asthma, was added. This medication contained ephedrine, a heart stimulant. A volunteer test subject then immediately drank the water containing the medication. Thirty minutes later, the other half of the microwaved water had a solution of Primatene added by a person in a different room, 50 feet away from the test subject, who was not aware of this happening. The test subject was being monitored by a device recording his heart rate. When the medication was added to the other half of the water solution, the heart rate of the test subject simultaneously "rapidly increased," for a period of four minutes, as if the test subject had directly been infused with more medication. "Biologically/chemically meaningful information can be transmitted through quantum entanglement," concluded the researchers. "Our findings also assist the establishment of a unified scientific framework for explaining many anomalous effects such as telepathy and homeopathy, if they do indeed exist, thus transforming these anomalous effects into the domains of conventional sciences."

"Enhanced Power within a Predicted Narrow Band of Theta Activity During Stimulation of Another By Circumcerebral Weak Magnetic Fields After Weekly Spatial Proximity: Evidence for Macroscopic Quantum Entanglement?" Persinger MA. Et al. *NeuroQuantology*. 2008 March.

A team of scientists at Canada's Behavioral Neuroscience and Biomolecular lab, University of Laurentian, recruited four pairs of strangers (four men, four women, between 19 and 24 years of age) and had them meet each other for one hour, twice a week, over a four-week period. The experiment consisted of having one person from each pair sit in a closed chamber, where they were exposed to six, five-minute sessions of magnetic fields. "Before the experiment began," wrote the researchers, "the stimulus person, to whom the fields were delivered, was told to imagine being in the other room with their partner and to imagine touching him or her." Seated in another room, the other member of the four pairs had their brains monitored. Each time the 'sender' received a dose of magnetic field exposure, the 'receiver' in another room also experienced changes in the temporal lobes of their brain, simultaneous with experiencing 'sensed presences' and emotional arousal. This experiment duplicated the results of a previous lab test that involved siblings, conducted by the same research team in 2003.

"Transatlantic Excess Brain Correlations Are Experimentally Produced by Persinger's Group." Hu H. Wu M. *Journal of Consciousness Exploration & Research.* 2015 September.

Psychologist Michael Persinger and his research team at Laurentian University, Canada, recruited five pairs of volunteers in 2015 and separated them by several thousand miles. They all sat in laboratories and wore identical brain devices that produced magnetic field sequences. When the magnetic field was pulsed in the brains of one set of volunteers, their partners across the Atlantic Ocean, several thousand miles away, simultaneously experienced reactions that were recorded in their right temporal brain lobes. These findings seem to represent further support for the idea of biological quantum entanglement.

"Physically disconnected non-diffusible cell-to-cell communication between neuroblastoma SH-SY5Y and DRG primary sensory neurons." Chaban VV. Et al. *Am J Tranl Res.* 2013.

Four scientists at UCLA's Geffen School of Medicine investigated non-traditional, yet physically connected pathways in cell-to-cell communication, using brain neuron cells. They wondered if these cells could communicate through "a higher level of non-linear communication," such as what happens with flocks of birds, or other self-organizing collective systems in nature. They divided up batches of neuron cells, called dorsal root ganglia neurons, into separate dish containers, "in a Faraday cage to protect neurons from electromagnetic influence" coming from the surrounding room. When one dish of cells was stimulated, the other dish of separated partner cells responded, indicating a previously unknown cell-to-cell signaling mechanism.

"New perspective in cell communication: Potential role of ultra-weak photon emission." Prasad A. Et al. *Journal of Photochemistry and Photobiology*. 2014.

In this review of studies, done by biophysics scientists based in Italy, Switzerland, and the Czech Republic, ultra-weak photons of light were assessed as a mechanism for cell-to-cell communication that is "1000 times lower than the sensitivity of the human eye." Terminologies in use to describe the phenomenon include: biophoton emission, biological chemiluminescence, or autoluminescence. Organisms that emit spontaneous ultra-weak photons are not engaging in luminescence because there isn't any photoexcitation going on. Stress conditions in plants, such as temperature fluctuations and pathogen infection, have been shown in experiments to produce ultra-weak photon emissions. Other research on human hands has shown "that both palmar and dorsal side of the hands emits the same number of photons, which is not gender specific, and the emission was recorded in the visible region of the spectrum." Other experiments showed that ultra-weak photon emission is dependent on the thickness of the skin. "Recently experiments to evaluate if two different cell populations influence each other when kept in close proximity, utilizing fibroblast and endothelial cells, were performed. The two cultures were separated by polystyrene petri dishes transparent… and a strong influence of one over the other…was observed." The origin and mechanism of ultra-weak photon emission is not clearly understood.

"The Efficacy of 'Distant Healing': A Systematic Review of Randomized Trials." Astin JA. Et al. *Annals of Internal Medicine*. 2000.

In a systematic review of the available study data, examining the effectiveness of Therapeutic Touch, mental healing, and distant healing prayer practices, British and American scientists looked at the results from 23 clinical trials involving 2,774 patients. Five studies examined prayer as a distant healing intervention; 11 assessed noncontact Therapeutic Touch; and 7 looked at other forms of distant healing. Of those studies, 57% "yielded statistically significant treatment effects."

"The effects of distant healing performed by a spiritual healer on chronic pain: a randomized controlled trial." Tsubono K. Et al. Altern. *Ther. Health Med.* 2009 May.

Three chronic pain specialists recruited 17 volunteers, all suffering from chronic pain conditions following injury or surgery. Subjects were randomly assigned to a treatment or control group. The treatment involved a 20-minute group meditation led by a professional Japanese distant healer. After the session, the healer flew back to Japan. Over the next two months, members of the treatment group meditated for 20 minutes each day, as the healer in Japan did his distant healing practice with them in mind. "Comparison of pretreatment and posttreatment visual analog scale indicated a slightly significant effect of distant healing" on a Pain Rating index, according to the study authors. Another measure, The Present Pain Intensity Scale, "showed significant improvement in the treatment group compared to the control group."

"Seeds induced to germinate rapidly by mentally projected 'qi energy' are apparently genetically altered." Bai F. Et al. *American Journal of Chinese Medicine*. 2000.

A practitioner of Waiqi, which is a form of qigong, using qi energy, as identified in traditional Chinese medicine, was tested for her ability to project qi energy to influence seed growth. Chulin Sun, by name, was a member of the Chinese Somatic Science Research Institute, who had been tested 180 times previously at university and science research institutes in China, Hong Kong, Taiwan, Japan, and Thailand. In this experiment, conducted by a team of 11 researchers, she was asked to 'treat' groups of wheat and pea seeds using her mentally-projected qi energy. Twenty wheat and pea seeds were placed in small containers and treated by Chulin Sun for about 20 minutes; whereas an equal number of seeds in a control group were germinated naturally in an incubator. Small amounts of DNA were extracted from both the experimental and control groups of seeds. The application of qi had "increased the rate of cellular growth and division, hundreds of times, compared to the control seeds," reported the research team. Changes were also observed in the structure of DNA taken from the experimental group of seeds.

"Modulation of germination and growth by plants by meditation." Haid M. Et al. *American Journal of Chinese Medicine*. 2001.

At Northwestern University Medical School, a series of double-blind experiments were conducted using meditators, to see if meditating on a glass of water could affect the germination of seeds when the water was added. The meditation 'treated' water was added to green pea and wheat seeds. In the case of the green pea seeds, for instance, the germination of 504 seeds receiving the treated water was 60.3%, compared to 51.8%

for the 504 control seeds. This difference was considered statistically significant.

"Non-Chemical Distant Cellular Interactions as a potential confounder of cell biology experiments." Farhadi A. *Frontiers in Physiology.* 2014 October.

In this review of research on non-chemical, distant cellular interactions, electromagnetic waves are identified as having the most experimental support to explain non-chemical distant cellular interactions. While there is "no question that cells can be affected by electromagnetic waves over a wide range of electromagnetic frequencies," including the "specialized, light-detecting cells in our body such as retinal, and pineal cells," this "phenomenon is still speculative" when it comes to the precise mechanism and how it works. "There is no solid scientific data to show which range or types of electromagnetic waves are being used." However, once the mechanism for these cellular interactions is identified, "this new information will introduce a revolutionary mechanism to the field of cellular biology."

"The Theory and Practice of Syntonic Phototherapy: A Review." Wallace LB. *Optometry & Vision Development.* 2009.

Syntonic Optometry holds that "specific light frequencies entering the eye can balance the autonomic and endocrine systems," another example of how light affects physiology.

"The application of colored light for healing dates back to the earliest times of recorded history, including Egyptian and Mayan civilizations. The modern use of color therapy can be found in the works of Edwin Babbitt, M.D., Carl Loeb, M.D.," pioneers in the late 1800s and early 1900s, who "used colored light shown directly on the body to treat hundreds of physical and psychological conditions."

"The breakthrough research in the ocular application of specific frequencies of light was conducted by Harry Reilly Spitler, M.D., who published his seminal work, The Syntonic Principle, in 1941. Spitler was the first to detail the biology of the non-optic tract showing ocular light stimulation results in changing the physiology of the thalamus, hypothalamus and pituitary gland. Syntonics, derived from the word 'syntony', means to bring into balance, specifically the autonomics and endocrine systems which serve as the major support neurologically to vision. Spitler concluded that imbalances in the nervous and hormonal systems caused many bodily, mental/emotional, and visual ailments. Spitler detailed how specific light frequencies effect cell biology, inherent electrical systems in the eye and brain, eye physiology, ocular functions, and emotional centers. This also includes light frequencies having the ability to affect EEG patterns. It is believed that certain color frequencies can build or discharge electrical potentials between cell walls and between organs such as the brain and liver."

"The syntonic model suggests that low energy/long wave-length (red) visible light stimulates the sympathetic nervous system, middle frequencies like green light balances physiology, and high energy/short wave light (blue) activates the parasympathetic nervous systems…The physiological model presented by Spitler was ahead of its time. It was later fully documented by Fritz Hollwich, M.D., in his text, The Influence of Ocular Light Perception on Metabolism in Man and Animal, in 1979."

"Tina Karu, a Russian biophysicist, has conducted much of the leading research in this area. Among many of her findings, she has demonstrated that coherent and non-coherent colored light can directly enhance cellular metabolism via the respiratory chain, cellular signaling, as well as ATP production through direct responses in the mitochondria, RNA and DNA synthesis. The field of biological utilization of lasers also illustrates how light can be used as treatment. Current research and various aspects of using light as therapy can be reviewed in the Journal of Biophotonics and on the web at http://www.worldlaserassociation.com.

"In his ground-breaking research, William Douglas, M.D., found that irradiating blood with ultraviolet light had profound effects on the immune and energy systems of the body. He found that drawing 1.5 ml of blood, irradiating it for 10 seconds and then injecting it back into the body would inactivate toxins, kill bacteria, increase oxygen content and cell function."

"In the fields of quantum biology and integrative biophysics a new paradigm is emerging that in part theorizes that light and electromagnetic fields are the energy and information organizers of all organic activity. A cell may have a hundred thousand reactions occurring per second. How does the body coordinate all these biological events to create the symphony of parts which make us whole? This is beyond the scope of traditional biochemical models. It has been shown that when blood is exposed to light and color, it changes its crystalline structure becoming less or more organized depending on the coherence and quality of the irradiation. Water itself has a charge density plasma that creates direct currents that are self-organizing, internally generated, and very sensitive to the environment's electromagnetic fields. The charge density changes its positive and negative charges with anabolic and catabolic actions in the body. This may be another communication system that relies on local and non-local energy such as light from the environment."

"Presently there are many healing professions that utilize light and color. Low-power lasers are used by physiotherapists for acute and chronic musculoskeletal injuries, by dentists to treat inflamed oral tissues, and by dermatologists for pain, ulcers, burns and dermatitis. Rheumatologists use cool lasers for pain and inflammation. Color is applied to various points in the body corresponding to acupuncture and muscle trigger points. The most well-known applications are in the field of psychiatry where light is used to treat seasonal affective disorder. A field of acupuncture has been created called color puncture, where needles have been replaced by small beams of different colors on the acupuncture points."

"The Effect of 'Healing with Intent' on Pepsin Enzyme Activity." Bunnell T. *Journal of Scientific Exploration.* 1999.

A British study at the School of Health, University of Hull, examined whether 'healing with intent' (Reiki, therapeutic touch, etc.) could influence pepsin enzyme activity "by affecting the state of ionization of the side-chains of amino acid residues at the active site." Altogether, 20 separate trials were conducted, measuring the reaction rates of enzyme samples isolated in test tubes and exposed to 'healing intent energy' directed at the tubes by energy practitioners. Reaction rates in the treated versus untreated enzyme samples were "significantly greater," concluded the study, which the author speculated was the result of a "pulsing magnetic field emitted from the hands during the delivery of healing with intent."

"Evidence for Correlations Between Distant Intentionality and Brain Function in Recipients: A Functional Magnetic Resonance Imaging Analysis." Achterberg J. Et al. *The Journal of Alternative and Complementary Medicine.* 2005.

Eleven energy practitioners who claimed to do healing at a distance were recruited for this experiment, which was conducted by a team of six scientists, including one from Stanford University Medical Center. The practitioners represented numerous energy channeling traditions—Healing Touch, Reiki, traditional Hawaiian *pule*, Qigong, and others. Each study volunteer selected a person they felt connected to, as a 'receiver' of the distant intentionality. The receivers were hooked up to MRI brain scanners while isolated from all sensory contact with the 'senders' of distant intentionality (DI), who were in electromagnetically shielded control rooms. At random two-minute intervals, senders sent their intentions to the receivers, who were completely unaware of the timing. Three areas of the brains of receivers were found to be activated when the senders were sending remotely—the anterior and middle cingulated area (concerned with executive control and decision-making), precuneus (part of a neural network involved with self-reflection), and the frontal lobe area (involved with information processing). "Overall," wrote the study authors, "the results show significant activation of brain regions coincident with distant intentionality intervals. Given that there are no known biological processes that can account for the significant effect of the DI protocol, the results of this study may be interpreted as consistent with the idea of entanglement in quantum mechanics theory."

"Can We Help Just by Good Intentions? A Meta-Analysis of Experiments on Distant Intention Effects." Schmidt S. *The Journal of Alternative and Complementary Medicine.* 2012.

A meta-analysis was conducted among 11 studies examining "whether a positive distant intention can be related to some outcome in a target person." A meta-analysis is a statistical technique for combining the findings from multiple independent studies on a topic to determine a common trend or truth. "The hypothesis of the positive effect of benevolent intentions is supported by the data presented," the meta-analysis determined. "It is concluded that especially the intentional aspect may be responsible for these unorthodox findings. These findings may have implications for distant healing research and health care as well as for meditation performance."

"Therapeutic Touch Stimulates the Proliferation of Human Cells in Culture." Gronowicz GA. Et al. *The Journal of Alternative and Complementary Medicine.* 2008.

Five scientists with the University of Connecticut Health Center tested the effects of Therapeutic Touch (TT) on the proliferation of normal human cells, in culture, that included neonatal foreskin fibroblasts cultures, and cells taken from tendons and bones. Three TT practitioners, each a registered nurse, were recruited who applied two 10-minute TT treatments per week, which "significantly stimulated proliferation in all cell types," compared to untreated cells. The TT practitioners held their hands about 10 inches away from the specimens while directing positive intentions through the hands. "The finding that all three cell types responded to two TT treatments a week for 2 weeks suggests that there is a threshold for TT treatments that affects proliferation in multiple cell types and that there may be common factors involved in proliferation that are the target for energy treatments," wrote the study authors.

"Towards Explaining Anomalously Large Body Voltage Surges on Exceptional Subjects." Tiller WA. Et al. *Journal of Scientific Exploration.* 1995.

And, "Anomalous electrostatic phenomena in exceptional subjects." Green EE. Et al. *Subtle Energies.* 1991.

Discussion is given about Elmer Green's 1991 findings "in a copperwall laboratory experiment with 9 'exceptional' subjects, experienced therapeutic touch TT therapists: 6 women and 3 men. During TT session with patients, these therapists produced large anomalous body potential surges (measured at an ear lobe) ranging from -4 V to -190 V, lasting from approximately 0.5 s to 12.5 s, measured with an electrometer. On average, these electrical signals were approximately 103 times larger than psychophysiologic galvanic skin potential changes associated with emotional responses, 105 times larger than electrocardiographic voltages. On the surrounding four copper walls, voltage signals were recorded in synchrony with the therapist's surge of body potential."

"It appears from the data of Green et al. that the training and practice involved in TT develops in the healer a somewhat automatic internal power buildup at subtle levels of the body that discharges periodically and generates a very large electrical voltage pulse in the physical body. When the healer is intentionally healing, these internal voltage surges increase in both frequency and magnitude."

"Human Consciousness Influence on Water Structure." Pyatnitsky LN. Fonkin VA. *Journal of Scientific Exploration.* 1995.

To examine whether directed human intentions can alter the structure of water, Russian scientists did more than 2,000 'runs,' or tests, involving 15 persons acting as 'operators.' Water from an urban water supply was used, kept at a constant temperature, and monitored for any changes in conductivity, surface tension, elasticity, density, refractivity, and light polarization. "Alterations of scattered light intensity, correlated with an operator's intention, sometimes exceeded factors of 10 to 1,000 the statistical variances observed before or after operator interaction," concluded the study authors. "Such effects have been demonstrated by several operators, and appear to be operator-specific, although enhanceable by training. Though we have no explanation of the phenomenon, the data represented in this paper would seem to indicate that some human operators can produce a consciousness-related influence on water structure."

"Towards a Quantitative Model of Both Local and Non-Local Energetic/ Information Healing." Tiller WA. *The International Journal of Healing and Caring*. 2003 May.

"Unusually large electromagnetic pulses were observed in the body of an expert healer, ranging from 30 volts to 300 volts, astoundingly, about 100,000 times normal. These voltage pulses correlated with external pulses ranging from 1 to 5 volts, measured at a distance of several feet from the healer's body. Tiller's model proposes that these effects draw upon energy available to highly self-regulated people, emerging from a condition of higher than usual symmetry with information waves in the vacuum, based on magnetic processes."

"In Vitro effect of Reiki Treatment on Bacterial Cultures: Role of Experimental Context and Practitioner Well-Being." Rubik B. Schwartz GE. Et al. *The Journal of Alternative and Complementary Medicine*. 2006.

Can bacteria that has been heat-shocked, recover by exposure to Reiki treatments? To answer that question, three researchers associated with the University of Arizona, cultures of Escherichia coli K12 bacteria were heat shocked, and then given 15 minutes of Reiki hands treatment by practitioners. "Reiki treated cultures overall exhibited significantly more bacteria than controls," the study concluded. Just as interesting, practitioners with a higher level of well-being had greater success in reviving the bacteria, compared to controls. Lower emotional well-being by practitioners during treatments resulted in fewer surviving bacteria.

"Measuring Effects of Music, Noise, and Healing Energy Using a Seed Germination Bioassay." Creath K. Schwartz GE. *The Journal of Alternative and Complementary Medicine*. 2004.

The effects of healing energy, noise, and music were tested on the germination of okra and zucchini seeds. A biofield energy practitioner directed healing intention for 15-20 minutes, every 12 hours, at the seeds and had "a significant effect" in accelerating the germinating of the seeds, compared to untreated control seeds. Musical sounds, but not noise, also exerted effects on the speed of seed growth.

INDEX

BIBLIOGRAPHY

Ashcroft, Frances. *The Spark of Life: Electricity in the Human Body.* 2012: W.W. Norton.

Becker, Robert O. *The Body Electric: Electromagnetism and the Foundation of Life,* 1985: William Morrow.

Benor, Daniel J. *Consciousness Bioenergy and Healing,* 2004, Wholistic Healing Publications.

Benson, Herbert, 1996. *Timeless Healing: The Power and Biology of Belief.* New York: Scribners.

Bengston, William, Ph.D. *The Energy Cure: Unraveling the Mystery of Hands-On-Healing.* 2010: Sounds True.

Cousins, Norman. 1981. *Anatomy of an Illness.* New York: Bantam

Cousins, Norman. 1989. *Biology of Hope.* New York: Dutton

Dossey, Larry. *One Mind: How Our Individual Mind Is Part of a Greater Consciousness and Why It Matters,* 2014, Hay House

Dossey, Larry. *Healing Words: The Power of Prayer and the Practice of Medicine,* 1995.HarperOne

Dossey, Larry. *Healing Beyond the Body: Medicine and the Infinite Reach of the Mind.* 2003, Shambhala

Gerber, Richard. *Vibrational Medicine: The Handbook of Subtle-Energy Therapies,* 2001, Bear & Company

Gynn, Graham. *Return to the Brain of Eden.* 2007, Inner Traditions

Hunt, Valerie, Ph.D. *Infinite Mind: Science of the Human Vibrations and Consciousness,* 1989: Malibu Publishing.

McFadden, Johnjoe, and Al-Khalili, Jim. *Life on the Edge: The Coming Age of Quantum Biology.* 2014: Crown.

Oschman, James. *Energy Medicine in Therapeutics and Human Performance,* 2003, Butterworth Heinemann.

Pearsall, Paul. 1998. *The Heart's Code.* New York: Random House

Pearsall, Paul. 1996. *The Pleasure Principle.* Alameda, CA: Hunter House

Pert, Candace 1997. *Molecules of Emotion.* New York: Touchstone.

Peirce, Penney. *Frequency: The Power of Personal Vibration.* 2009: Atria.

Schwartz, Gary, Ph.D. *The Energy Experiments: Science Reveals Our Natural Power to Heal.* 2008: Atria.

Tiller, William A., Ph.D. *Psychoenergetic Science: A Second Copernican-Style Revolution.* 2007: Pavior Publishing.

ABOUT THE AUTHOR

Brian Clement, PhD., NMD., L.N., has spearheaded the international progressive health movement for more than five decades. He is the Co-Director, along with his wife Anna Maria, of the renowned Hippocrates Health Institute (HHI), West Palm Beach, Florida (U.S.A.). HHI is the world's foremost complementary residential health center and is known for its innovative educational programs. It has been helping people to help themselves since 1956 in Boston, relocating to Florida in 1986. There, Clement and the Institute have spearheaded major trends in the field of natural health over the decades.

Over the last half-century, he and his team have pioneered clinical research and training in disease prevention involving hundreds of thousands of participants. This has given Clement a privileged insight into the lifestyle required to prevent disease, enhance longevity, and maintain vitality. These findings have provided the basis for Hippocrates' progressive, state-of-the-art treatments and protocols for health maintenance and recovery – their Life Transformation Program. More than 600,000 people from over 70 countries have been guests in its Life Transformation Program, and thousands more have become certified Hippocrates Health Educators.

Along with his wife, Anna Maria Gahns-Clement, Ph.D., L.N., Brian Clement co-directs the Hippocrates Health Institute. In addition to his research studies, Clement conducts dozens of conferences worldwide each year on attaining health and creating longevity, giving humanity a roadmap for redirecting, enriching, and extending their lives.

A licensed nutritionist, Brian Clement is a graduate of the University of Science, Arts, and Technology where he earned his Ph.D.

Clement is the author or co-author of more than 20 books, including:

Living Foods for Optimum Health, 1998, Harmony.

Hippocrates LifeForce, 2007, Healthy Living Publications (Cornell University nutritional biochemist Dr. Colin Campbell called this book, in his Preface to it, "One of the most important books ever written on nutrition."

Supplements Exposed, 2009, New Page Books.

Man-opause, 2012, Roman & Littlefield.

REFERENCES

[1] Duncan, F., Que, E., Zhang, N. et al. The zinc spark is an inorganic signature of human egg activation. Sci Rep 6, 24737 (2016). https://doi.org/10.1038/srep24737

[2] Grynberg, M., et al. "First Birth Achieved After Fertility Preservation Using Vitrification of In Vitro Matured Oocytes in a Woman with Breast Cancer." *Annals of Oncology*, vol. 31, no. 4, Apr. 2020, pp. 541-542, https://doi.org/10.1016/j.annonc.2020.01.005.

[3] An, Daniel, Krzysztof A. Meissner, Paweł Nurowski, and Roger Penrose. "Apparent Evidence for Hawking Points in the CMB Sky." *Monthly Notices of the Royal Astronomical Society*, vol. 495, no. 3, July 2020, pp. 3403-3408, https://doi.org/10.1093/mnras/staa1343.

[4] Planck, Max. *The Theory of Heat Radiation.* Translated by Morton Masius, Project Gutenberg, 18 June 2012, https://www.yaaka.cc/wp-content/uploads/2018/02/the-theory-of-heat-radiation.pdf. Accessed 3 Oct. 2024.

[5] "Einstein and the Photoelectric Effect." *APS News | This Month in Physics History*, American Physical Society, 1 Jan. 2005, https://www.aps.org/apsnews/2005/01/einstein-photoelectric-effect. Accessed 3 Oct. 2024.

[6] "The Nobel Prize in Physics 1921." *NobelPrize.org*, Nobel Prize Outreach AB, https://www.nobelprize.org/prizes/physics/1921/summary/. Accessed 3 Oct. 2024.

[7] Britannica, The Editors of Encyclopaedia. "Schrödinger equation." Encyclopedia Britannica, 13 Sep. 2024, https://www.britannica.com/science/Schrodinger-equation. Accessed 3 October 2024.

[8] Britannica, The Editors of Encyclopaedia. "uncertainty principle." Encyclopedia Britannica, 16 Aug. 2024, https://www.britannica.com/science/uncertainty-principle. Accessed 3 October 2024.

[9] "Valerie V. Hunt 1916-2014." *ValerieVHunt.com*, http://valerievhunt.com/ValerieVHunt.com/Valerie_Hunt_EdD.html. Accessed 3 Oct. 2024.

[10] Lewerenz, Hans-Joachim. *Photons in natural and life sciences: an interdisciplinary approach.* Vol. 157. Springer, 2013.

[11] Shams, Muhammad, et al. "The Quantum-Medical Nexus: Understanding the Impact of Quantum Technologies on Healthcare." *Cureus*, vol. 15, no. 10, 31 Oct. 2023, e48077, https://doi.org/10.7759/cureus.48077. Accessed 3 Oct. 2024.

[12] "Notable Living Contemporary Teachers: Valerie Hunt Ed.D." *Awaken*, Nov. 2022, https://awaken.com/2022/11/valerie-hunt/. Accessed 3 Oct. 2024.

[13] Bynum, William. "Singing the Body Electric." *The Wall Street Journal*, 28 Sept. 2012, 3:37 p.m. ET, https://www.wsj.com/articles/SB1000087 23963904448127045776097908480493320. Accessed 3 Oct. 2024.

[14] Evans, G. W. (1982). *Environmental stress*. Cambridge University Press.

[15] "How We Know the Universe Is 13.8 Billion Years Old." *Big Think,* 8 Apr. 2024, https://bigthink.com/starts-with-a-bang/universe-13-8-billion-years-old/. Accessed 3 Oct. 2024.

[16] Harari, Yuval N. Sapiens: A Brief History of Humankind. New York: Harper, 2015.

[17] Stein, Vicky, and Daisy Dobrijevic. "Do Parallel Universes Exist? We Might Live in a Multiverse." *Space.com,* 3 Nov. 2021. Accessed 3 Oct. 2024, https://web.archive.org/web/20211003032728/https://www.space.com/32728-parallel-universes.html

[18] Planck, Max. "Zur Theorie des Gesetzes der Energieverteilung im Normalspektrum." *Annalen der Physik*, vol. 309, no. 3, 1900, pp. 553-563.

[19] Calaprice, Alice. *The Ultimate Quotable Einstein*. Princeton University Press, 2011.

[20] Nave, R. "Composition of the Sun." *HyperPhysics*, Georgia State University, http://hyperphysics.phy-astr.gsu.edu/hbase/Tables/suncomp.html.

[21] Britannica, The Editors of Encyclopaedia. "bremsstrahlung." Encyclopedia Britannica, 12 May. 2023, https://www.britannica.com/science/bremsstrahlung. Accessed 3 October 2024.

[22] Sharp, Tim, and Ailsa Harvey. "What Is the Sun Made Of?" *Space.com*, 27 Jan. 2022, retrieved from https://www.space.com/17170-what-is-the-sun-made-of.html

[23] Norris, Jeffrey. "Cell Phones Pose Health Risks, Says Devra Davis at UCSF Seminar." *University of California San Francisco*, https://www.ucsf.edu/news/2010/10/103624/cell-phones-pose-health-risks-says-devra-davis-ucsf-seminar. Accessed 3 Oct. 2024.

[24] Belkaid, Y., & Hand, T. W. (2014). Role of the Microbiota in Immunity and Inflammation. *Cell*, 157(1), 121–141. DOI: 10.1016/j.cell.2014.03.011.

[25] **Owen, B., Hatala, A., Hylton, K., & Harris, N. (2021).** Traditional Indigenous Medicine in North America: A scoping review. *PLOS ONE, 16*(8), e0237531. 10.1371/journal.pone.0237531

[26] Sirisha, D., et al. "Brain to Brain Communication: A Study on Future Technology." *Journal of Emerging Technologies and Innovative Research (JETIR)*, vol. 6, no. 3, Mar. 2019, pp. 591-597, https://www.jetir.org/papers/JETIR1903685.pdf

[27] Ferguson-Smith AC, Patti ME. 2011. You are what your dad ate. Cell Metab 13(2):115117, PMID: 21284975, 10.1016/j.cmet.2011.01.011.

[28] Braun JM, Messerlian C, Hauser R. 2017. Fathers matter: why it's time to consider the impact of paternal environmental exposures on children's health. Curr Epidemiol Rep 4(1):46–55, PMID: 28848695, 10.1007/s40471-017-0098-8.

[29] Rando OJ. 2012. Daddy issues: paternal effects on phenotype. Cell 151(4):702–708, PMID: 23141533, 10.1016/j.cell.2012.10.020.

[30] Britannica, The Editors of Encyclopaedia. "dowsing." Encyclopedia Britannica, 27 Sep. 2024, https://www.britannica.com/topic/dowsing.

[31] West, Michael. *Investigation of Viktor Schauberger's Vortex Engine*. B.Sc. Thesis, School of Engineering, The University of Queensland, 2005, https://doi.org/10.14264/300139.

[32] Britannica, The Editors of Encyclopaedia. "extrasensory perception." Encyclopedia Britannica, 25 May. 2024, https://www.britannica.com/topic/extrasensory-perception. Accessed 2 October 2024.

[33] Tammet, Daniel. *Daniel Tammet Official Website*, http://danieltammet.net/. Accessed 10 Sep. 2024.

[34] "FDA Approves Pill with Sensor That Digitally Tracks if Patients Have Ingested Their Medication." *FDA News Release*, 13 Nov. 2017, https://www.fda.gov/news-events/press-announcements/fda-approves-pill-sensor-digitally-tracks-if-patients-have-ingested-their-medication. Accessed 10 Sept. 2024.

[35] **Lieberman, J.** (1991). *Light: Medicine of the Future: How We Can Use It to Heal Ourselves Now*. Bear & Company.

[36] **Rauscher, F. H., Shaw, G. L., & Ky, K. N.** (1993). Music and spatial task performance. Nature, 365(6447), 611. https://doi.org/10.1038/365611a0

[37] *Wholetones*. https://wholetones.com/?srsltid=AfmBOoq_xPmGGmffsFYNrkPfh5L7pf02EIeS8qqWZvWa0Bj_hI6EbphX. Accessed 3 Oct. 2024.

[38] Hirshberg, C. (2011, April 5). *Spontaneous remission: The spectrum of self-repair*. The Human Mind. Retrieved from https://humanmind overmatter.blogspot.com/2011/04/spontaneous-remission.html

[39] *Pure Synergy*. "Our Founder." https://thesynergycompany.com/pages/our-founder?srsltid=AfmBOooYXep7FXLv1V3uTR2UU6BfgjMZey1w-9Bbk7nuD1tVdYrNEwq7. Accessed 3 Oct. 2024.

[40] Dawson, Edgar G., M.D. *Health Central*, https://www.healthcentral.com/author/edgar-g-dawson. Accessed 25 Sept. 2024.

[41] Cook, Lana. *Altered States: The American Psychedelic Aesthetic*. Dissertation, Northeastern University, 2014, https://repository.library.northeastern.edu/files/neu:336751/fulltext.pdf. Accessed 3 Oct. 2024.

[42] *Father Brown The Detective*. Directed by Robert Hamer, performances by Alec Guinness, Joan Greenwood, and Peter Finch, Facet Prods, 1954. *Archive.org*, https://archive.org/details/father-brown-the-detective-1954-mys.-detec.-alec-guiness. Accessed 3 Oct. 2024

[43] Newland, Constance A., pseud. *Myself and I*. Coward-McCann, 1962. *Archive.org*, https://archive.org/details/myself00newl. Accessed 3 Oct. 2024.

[44] Britannica, The Editors of Encyclopaedia. "parapsychology." Encyclopedia Britannica, 26 Jul. 2024, https://www.britannica.com/topic/parapsychology. Accessed 3 October 2024.

[45] Taff, Barry E. "Legacy's End: The Rise and Fall of the UCLA Parapsychology Lab." *The Teeming Brain*, 15 Nov. 2012, https://www.teemingbrain.com/2012/11/15/legacys-end-the-rise-and-fall-of-the-ucla-parapsychology-lab/. Accessed 3 Oct. 2024.

[46] Britannica, The Editors of Encyclopaedia. "qi." Encyclopedia Britannica, 21 Sep. 2024, https://www.britannica.com/topic/qi-Chinese-philosophy.

[47] Britannica, The Editors of Encyclopaedia. "prana." Encyclopedia Britannica, 2 Mar. 2015, https://www.britannica.com/topic/prana. Accessed 3 October 2024.

[48] "About Causalgia." *UCLA Health*, https://www.uclahealth.org/medical-services/neurosurgery/conditions-treated/causalgia#:~:text=Medical%20therapy%20is%20usually%20ineffective.

[49] "Mitchell May & The Synergy Story." *Moonflower Community Cooperative*, https://moonflower.coop/mitchell-may-the-synergy-story/.

[50] Schmidt, S. (2004). *Mindfulness and healing intention: Concepts, practice, and research evaluation. The Journal of Alternative and Complementary Medicine, 10*(Suppl 1), S-7–S-14. https://doi.org/10.1089/acm.2004.10.S-7

[51] O'Regan, B., & Hirshberg, C. (1993). *Spontaneous remission: An annotated bibliography.* Institute of Noetic Sciences. Retrieved from https://noetic.org/publication/spontaneous-remission-annotated-bibliography/

[52] Britannica, The Editors of Encyclopaedia. "Edgar Mitchell." Encyclopedia Britannica, 13 Sep. 2024, https://www.britannica.com/biography/Edgar-D-Mitchell. Accessed 3 October 2024.

[53] Turner, K. A. (2010). *Spontaneous remission of cancer: Theories from healers, physicians, and cancer survivors* (Doctoral dissertation). University of California, Berkeley. ProQuest Dissertations & Theses Global. (3444696).

[54] Schlitz, M. (1993). *Spontaneous remission: An annotated bibliography.* Institute of Noetic Sciences. Chapter 11: Remission of Infectious and Parasitic Diseases, p. 354. Retrieved from https://noetic.org/publication/spontaneous-remission-annotated-bibliography/

[55] Kassoff, A., & Welty, C. (1983). Spontaneous recovery phenomenon in the presumed ocular histoplasmosis syndrome. *International Ophthalmology Clinics, 23*(2), 105-112. Available at PubMed: https://pubmed.ncbi.nlm.nih.gov/6189797/

[56] Mac Manus, Michael P., et al. "Unexpected Long-Term Survival After Low-Dose Palliative Radiotherapy for Nonsmall Cell Lung Cancer." *Cancer,* vol. 106, no. 5, 23 Jan. 2006, https://doi.org/10.1002/cncr.21704.

[57] "Prof Michael MacManus." *Find an Expert,* University of Melbourne, https://findanexpert.unimelb.edu.au/profile/6157-michael-macmanus

[58] Mac Manus, M. P., Matthews, J. P., Wada, M., Wirth, A., Worotniuk, V., & Ball, D. L. (2006). Unexpected long-term survival after low-dose palliative radiotherapy for nonsmall cell lung cancer. *Cancer, 106*(5), 1110-1116. https://doi.org/10.1002/cncr.21704

[59] Vandenberg, L. N., Colborn, T., Hayes, T. B., Heindel, J. J., Jacobs, D. R., Jr., Lee, D.-H., Shioda, T., Soto, A. M., vom Saal, F. S., Welshons, W. V., et al. (2012). Hormones and endocrine-disrupting chemicals: Low-dose effects and nonmonotonic dose responses. *Endocrine Reviews, 33*(3), 378–455. https://doi.org/10.1210/er.2011-1050

[60] Einstein, A. (1905). *Does the inertia of a body depend upon its energy content? Annalen der Physik,* 323(13), 639-641. https://doi.org/10.1002/andp.19053231314

[61] Moga, M. M., & Zhou, D. (2008). Distant healing of small-sized tumors. *Journal of Scientific Exploration, 22*(3), 353-363. https://pubmed.ncbi.nlm.nih.gov/18564948/

[62] Moga, Margaret M. *ResearchGate,* https://www.researchgate.net/profile/Margaret-Moga.

[63] Britannica, The Editors of Encyclopaedia. "moxibustion." Encyclopedia Britannica, 16 Jan. 2022, https://www.britannica.com/science/moxa-treatment. Accessed 25 September 2024.

[64] "The Role of Qi and Meridians." *Britannica,* https://www.britannica.com/science/traditional-Chinese-medicine.

[65] Yang, L., Yong, L., Zhu, X. et al. Disease progression model of 4T1 metastatic breast cancer. *J Pharmacokinet Pharmacodyn* 47, 105–116 (2020). https://doi.org/10.1007/s10928-020-09673-5

[66] Bengston, W. F., & Moga, M. (2007). Resonance, placebo effects, and type II errors: Some implications from healing research for experimental methods. *Journal of Alternative and Complementary Medicine, 13*(3), 317-327. https://doi.org/10.1089/acm.2007.6300.

[67] Rubik, B., Muehsam, D., Hammerschlag, R., & Jain, S. (2015). Biofield science and healing: History, terminology, and concepts. *Global Advances in Health and Medicine, 4*(Suppl), 8–14. https://doi.org/10.7453/gahmj.2015.038.suppl.

[68] Bengston, W. F., & Krinsley, D. (2000). The effect of the "laying on of hands" on transplanted breast cancer in mice. *Journal of Scientific Exploration, 14*(3), 353-364. Available at: https://journalofscientificexploration.org/index.php/jse/article/view/2837/1831.

[69] Grad, B., Cadoret, R. J., & Paul, G. I. (1961). The influence of an unorthodox method of treatment on wound healing in mice. *International Journal of Parapsychology, 3*(2), 5-24.

[70] "Medicine Ways: Traditional Healers and Healing." *Native Voices,* U.S. National Library of Medicine, https://www.nlm.nih.gov/nativevoices/exhibition/healing-ways/medicine-ways/key-role-of-ceremony.html#:~:text=Traditional%20healing%20ceremonies%20promote%20wellness,a%20variety%20of%20sacred%20objects.

[71] Kleisiaris CF, Sfakianakis C, Papathanasiou IV. Health care practices in ancient Greece: The Hippocratic ideal. J Med Ethics Hist Med. 2014 Mar 15;7:6. PMID: 25512827; PMCID: PMC4263393.

[72] Lanska, D., & Sechenov, I. M. (2007). **Franz Anton Mesmer and the Rise and Fall of Animal Magnetism: Dramatic Cures, Controversy, and Ultimately a Triumph for the Scientific Method.** In *Brain, Mind and Medicine: Essays in Eighteenth-Century Neuroscience* (pp. 301-320). Springer. Available at ResearchGate.

[73] Britannica, The Editors of Encyclopaedia. "Phineas Parkhurst Quimby." Encyclopedia Britannica, 3 Apr. 2024, https://www.britannica.com/biography/Phineas-Parkhurst-Quimby. Accessed 6 September 2024.

[74] Eddy, Mary Baker. *Science and Health with Key to the Scriptures. 1875. Christian Science,* https://www.christianscience.com/the-christian-science-pastor/science-and-health.

[75] Twain, M. (Samuel Clemens). (2006). **Christian Science**. Project Gutenberg. https://www.gutenberg.org/ebooks/3187

[76] Sportelli L. The Discovery, Development and Current Status of the Chiropractic Profession. Integr Med (Encinitas). 2019 Dec;18(6):20-22. PMID: 32549852; PMCID: PMC7238904.

[77] Holmes, E. S. (1938). *The Science of Mind.* TarcherPerigee.

[78] Britannica, The Editors of Encyclopaedia. "Religious Science." Encyclopedia Britannica, 7 Feb. 2014, https://www.britannica.com/topic/Religious-Science. Accessed 6 September 2024.

[79] "History." *UCLA Semel Institute,* https://www.semel.ucla.edu/cousins/history.

[80] "Faith, Hands and Auras." (1972, November 27). *Time.* https://content.time.com/time/subscriber/article/0,33009,906598-1,00.html

[81] Schwartz, G. E., & Simon, W. L. (2008). *The Energy Healing Experiments: Science Reveals Our Natural Power to Heal.* Foreword by Richard Carmona. Atria Books.

[82] Dossey, L. (2001, June 16). *Spirituality, Science and the Medical Arts* [Keynote address]. ISSSEEM Eleventh Annual Conference.

[83] Dossey, L. (2002). How Healing Happens: Exploring the Nonlocal Gap. *Alternative Therapies in Health and Medicine,* Modified from a paper presented at "Bridging Worlds and Filling Gaps in the Science of Spiritual Healing," Conference on the Big Island, November 29-December 4, 2001, Keauhou Beach Resort, Kona, Hawaii.

[84] Orloff, J. (2017). *The Empath's Survival Guide: Life Strategies for Sensitive People* (First Edition). Sounds True. ISBN-10: 1622036573, ISBN-13: 978-1622036578.

[85] Peres, A. (2002). *Quantum Theory: Concepts and Methods.* Springer.

[86] Idels, M. (2024). *Nuclear Topology and the Blueprint of Matter.* Independently published. ISBN-13: 979-8323217267.

[87] Merali, Z. Not-quite-so elementary, my dear electron. *Nature* (2012). https://doi.org/10.1038/nature.2012.10471

[88] Ashcroft, F. (2012). *The Spark of Life: Electricity in the Human Body* (Illustrated edition). W. W. Norton & Company. ISBN-13: 978-0393078039.

[89] Hille, B. (2001). *Ion Channels of Excitable Membranes* (3rd ed.). Sinauer Associates.

[90] Guyton, A. C., & Hall, J. E. (2016). *Guyton and Hall Textbook of Medical Physiology* (13th ed.). Elsevier.

[91] Light GA, Williams LE, Minow F, Sprock J, Rissling A, Sharp R, Swerdlow NR, Braff DL. Electroencephalography (EEG) and event-related potentials (ERPs) with human participants. Curr Protoc Neurosci. 2010 Jul;Chapter 6:Unit 6.25.1-24. doi: 10.1002/0471142301.ns0625s52. PMID: 20578033; PMCID: PMC2909037.

[92] Haddock, S. H. D., Moline, M. A., & Case, J. F. (2010). "Bioluminescence in the Sea." *Annual Review of Marine Science,* 2, 443-493.

[93] Shukla, Usha. "Mechanisms and Applications of Bioluminescence." *J. Pure Appl. Ind. PhysicsAn Int. Res. Journal* 8.1 (2018): 1-6. https://www.researchgate.net/profile/Usha-Shukla-3/publication/378495886_Mechanisms_and_Applications_of_Bioluminescence/links/65dd667fadf2362b635a2d11/Mechanisms-and-Applications-of-Bioluminescence.pdf

[94] Becker, R. O. (1st ed.). (1985). *The Body Electric: Electromagnetism and the Foundation of Life.* Avon.

[95] Moss, Thelma, and John Hubacher. "The nature of Kirlian photography-an international overview." *15th Intl Congress on High Speed Photography and Photonics.* Vol. 348. SPIE, 1983.

[96] Becker, Robert O., and Andrew A. Marino. *Electromagnetism & Life.* Cassandra, 1982. https://www.naturalheightgrowth.com/wp-content/uploads/2013/12/Electromagnetism-and-Life.pdf. Accessed Oct. 2024.

[97] Benor, D. J. (2004). *Consciousness, Bioenergy and Healing: Self-Healing and Energy Medicine for the 21st Century* (pp. 411-416). Wholistic Healing Publications.

[98] Hunt, V. V. (1996). *Infinite mind: Science of the human vibrations of consciousness.* Malibu Publishing Co.

[99] Awaken. (2021, November 4). *The Human Energy Field: Dr. Valerie Hunt Interview Pt 1.* Awaken. https://awaken.com/2021/11/the-human-energy-field-dr-valerie-hunt-interview-part-1/

[100] Levin, M. Revisiting Burr and Northrop's "The Electro-Dynamic Theory of Life" (1935). *Biol Theory* **15**, 83–90 (2020). https://doi.org/10.1007/s13752-020-00341-y

[101] Ravitz, L. J. (1962). History, measurement, and applicability of periodic changes in the electromagnetic field in health and disease. *Annals of the New York Academy of Sciences,* 98(4), 1144-1201. https://doi.org/10.1111/j.1749-6632.1962.tb30626.x

[102] Hippocrates Wellness. *We Are the Original Pioneers of Longevity.* YouTube, 5 Mar. 2024, https://www.youtube.com/watch?v=PQcIxrTfqNA. Accessed 2 Oct. 2024.

[103] "Bion Energy: The Rubber That Radiates Harmony." *Facts are Facts,* https://www.facts-are-facts.com/article/bion-energy-the-rubber-that-radiates-harmony.

[104] Raknes, O. (2004). *Wilhelm Reich and Orgonomy.* American College of Orgonomy.

[105] Reich, Wilhelm. *The Orgone Energy Accumulator: Its Scientific and Medical Use.* Orgone Institute Press, pp. 19-27.

[106] A. D. Yaghjian, "Power-energy & dispersion relations for diamagnetic media," 2009 IEEE Antennas and Propagation Society InternationalSymposium, North Charleston, SC, USA, 2009, pp. 1-4, doi: 10.1109/APS.2009.5172325. keywords: {Dispersion;Magnetic materials;Metamaterials;Bismuth;Magnetic fields;Electromagnetics; Kinetic theory;Potential energy;Charge carriers;Conducting materials}

[107] Britannica, The Editors of Encyclopaedia. "paramagnetism." Encyclopedia Britannica, 29 Aug. 2024, https://www.britannica.com/science/paramagnetism. Accessed 6 September 2024.

[108] BADAK, BHAURAO S., and AJAY A. GURJAR. "ANALYSIS OF PATTERNS OF HEALING SOUNDS USING CYMATICS."

[109] Shteynberg, G. (2024). The psychology of collective consciousness. *Journal of Consumer Psychology.* https://doi.org/10.1002/jcpy.1434

[110] Gray, R., & Liotta, R. (2012). PTSD extinction, reconsolidation, and the visual-kinesthetic dissociation protocol. *Traumatology,* 18, 3-16. https://doi.org/10.1177/1534765611431835

[111] Devaraj, B., Usa, M., & Inaba, H. (1997). Biophotons: Ultraweak light emission from living systems. *Current Opinion in Solid State and Materials Science,* 2(2), 188-193. https://doi.org/10.1016/S1359-0286(97)80064-2

[112] Kobayashi M, Kikuchi D, Okamura H (2009) Imaging of Ultraweak Spontaneous Photon Emission from Human Body Displaying Diurnal Rhythm. PLoS ONE 4(7): e6256. https://doi.org/10.1371/journal.pone.0006256

[113] Choi, Charles Q. "Strange! Humans Glow in Visible Light." *LiveScience,* special to *LiveScience.com,* 22 July 2009, 10:32 a.m. ET. *Yahoo News* Archived version, https://labs.eis.tohtech.ac.jp/kobayashi/Yahoo.USA-YahooNews-July22.pdf. Accessed 3 Oct. 2024.

[114] Niggli, H. J., et al. "Laser-Ultraviolet-A Induced Ultra Weak Photon Emission in Human Skin Cells: A Biphotonic Comparison Between Keratinocytes and Fibroblasts." *Indian Journal of Experimental Biology,* vol. 46, May 2008, pp. 358-363.

[115] Van Wijk, R., & Van Wijk, E. P. A. (2005). An introduction to human biophoton emission. *Forschende Komplementärmedizin / Research in Complementary Medicine,* 12(2), 77–83. https://doi.org/10.1159/000083763

[116] Schutgens, F. W., et al. "The Influence of Adaptogens on Ultraweak Biophoton Emission: A Pilot-Experiment." *Phytotherapy Research,* vol. 23, no. 8, Aug. 2009, pp. 1103-1108.

[117] Van Wijk, E., et al. "Anatomic Characterization of Human Ultra-Weak Photon Emission in Practitioners of Transcendental Meditation and Control Subjects." *Journal of Alternative and Complementary Medicine,* vol. 12, no. 1, 2006, pp. 31-38.

[118] Dotta, B. T., et al. "Increased Photon Emission from the Head While Imagining Light in the Dark is Correlated with Changes in Electroencephalographic Power: Support for Bokkon's Biphoton Hypothesis." *Neuroscience Letters,* vol. 513, no. 2, Apr. 2012, pp. 151-154.

[119] Van Wijk, R. V., et al. "Correlation Between Fluctuations in Human Ultra-Weak Photon Emission and EEG Alpha Rhythm." *NeuroQuantology,* vol. 6, no. 4, 2008.

[120] Cahn, B. R., & Polich, J. (2006). Meditation states and traits: EEG, ERP, and neuroimaging studies. *Psychological Bulletin,* 132(2), 180–211. https://doi.org/10.1037/0033-2909.132.2.180

[121] Lustenberger, C., et al. "Functional Role of Frontal Alpha Oscillations in Creativity." *Cortex,* vol. 67, June 2015, pp. 74-82.

[122] Jenkins, D. (2017). A new calm: A story of breakthrough neuroscience technology patented to quickly and naturally reduce stress and improve performance. *CRANIO®,* 35(5), 342. https://doi.or g/10.1080/08869634.2017.1355591

[123] Benford MS, Talnagi J, Doss DB, Boosey S, Arnold LE. Gamma radiation fluctuations during alternative healing therapy. Altern Ther Health Med. 1999 Jul;5(4):51-6. PMID: 10394674.

[124] Seto, A., Kusaka, C., Nakazato, S., et al. "Detection of Extraordinary Large Biomagnetic Fields Strength from Human Hand." *Acupuncture and Electro-Therapeutics Research, International Journal,* vol. 17, 1992, pp. 75-94.

[125] Niedermeyer, E., & da Silva, F. L. (2005). *Electroencephalography: Basic Principles, Clinical Applications, and Related Fields* (5th ed.). Lippincott Williams & Wilkins.

[126] Rubik, B., & Jabs, H. (2017). Effects of intention, energy healing, and mind-body states on biophoton emission. *Cosmos and History: The Journal of Natural and Social Philosophy,* 13(2), 227

[127] Gottlieb, R. "Scientific Findings About Light's Impact on Biology." *Journal of Optometric Phototherapy,* Apr. 2000, pp. 1-4.

[128] Felten, S. Y., & Felten, D. L. (1994). Neural-immune interactions. In F. E. Bloom (Ed.), *Progress in Brain Research: Neuroscience: From the Molecular to the Cognitive* (Vol. 100, pp. 157-162). Elsevier. https://doi.org/10.1016/S0079-6123(08)60781-5

[129] Crichton, M. (1989). *Travels*. Random House Publishing Group. ISBN 978-0345359322.

[130] Orloff, J. (2001). *Dr. Judith Orloff's Guide to Intuitive Healing: 5 Steps to Physical, Emotional, and Sexual Wellness.* Harmony/Rodale. ISBN 978-0609805134.

[131] Coulson, R. L., & LaSalle, J. M. (2018). *Epigenetics of circadian rhythms in imprinted neurodevelopmental disorders. Progress in Molecular Biology and Translational Science, 157,* 67-92. https://doi.org/10.1016/bs.pmbts.2017.11.023

[132] Liberman, J. (1990). *Light: Medicine of the future.* Bear & Company.

[133] Lieverse, R., Van Someren, E. J. W., Nielen, M. M. A., Uitdehaag, B. M. J., Smit, J. H., & Hoogendijk, W. J. G. (2011). Bright light treatment in elderly patients with nonseasonal major depressive disorder: A randomized placebo-controlled trial. *Archives of General Psychiatry, 68*(1), 61-70. https://doi.org/10.1001/archgenpsychiatry.2010.183

[134] Saputo, Len. "Dr. Saputo's Biography." *DoctorSaputo.com,* https://www.doctorsaputo.com/a/dr-saputo-s-biography. Accessed 3 Oct. 2024.

[135] Saputo, Len. "A Breakthrough in Using Light Therapy to Treat Neuropathies." *The Townsend Letter,* Nov. 2015, https://web.archive.org/web/20170616142224/http://townsendletter.com/Nov2015/break1115.html. Accessed 3 Oct. 2024.

[136] Sisken, B. F., Kanje, M., Lundborg, G., Herbst, E., & Kurtz, W. (1989). Stimulation of rat sciatic nerve regeneration with pulsed electromagnetic fields. *Brain Research, 485*(2), 309-316. https://doi.org/10.1016/0006-8993(89)90575-1

[137] David Cohen, Edward Givler; Magnetomyography: magnetic fields around the human body produced by skeletal muscles. *Appl. Phys. Lett.* 1 August 1972; 21 (3): 114–116. https://doi.org/10.1063/1.1654294

[138] Stone, R. (1999). *Polarity Therapy: The complete collected works (Vol. 1).* Book Publishing Company (TN).

[139] Pall, M.L. (2013), Electromagnetic fields act *via* activation of voltage-gated calcium channels to produce beneficial or adverse effects. J. Cell. Mol. Med., 17: 958-965. https://doi.org/10.1111/jcmm.12088

[140] Dean, K. L. (2004). Understanding the human biofield and its role in whole person healing. *Alternative and Complementary Therapies, 9*(3). https://doi.org/10.1089/107628003322017396

[141]Rastogi, R., Chaturvedi, D.K., Rajeshwari, T., Sagar, S., & Tandon, N. (2023). Mantra and Homa Therapy: Computational Analysis of Different Aspects to Benefit Mankind with HealthCare 4.0 and Industry 5.0 Approach. *International Journal of Applied Research on Public Health Management.* https://doi.org/10.4018/IJARPHM.315815

[142] Hunt, V. V. (1996). *Infinite mind: Science of the human vibrations of consciousness.* Malibu Publishing.

[143] National Research Council. (2011). *Toward precision medicine: Building a knowledge network for biomedical research and a new taxonomy of disease.* The National Academies Press. https://doi.org/10.17226/13284

[144] Rang, H. P., Dale, M. M., Ritter, J. M., Flower, R. J., & Henderson, G. (2011). *Rang & Dale's Pharmacology* (7th ed.). Elsevier Churchill Livingstone.

[145] Levin, J. (2010). *Energy Healers: Who They Are and What They Do.* Institute for Studies of Religion, Baylor University.

[146] Howick J, Moscrop A, Mebius A, et al. Effects of empathic and positive communication in healthcare consultations: a systematic review and meta-analysis. Journal of the Royal Society of Medicine. 2018;111(7):240-252. doi:10.1177/0141076818769477

[147] Quest, P., & Roberts, K. (2010). *The Reiki Manual: A Training Guide for Reiki Students, Practitioners, and Masters.* TarcherPerigee.

[148] Creath, K., & Schwartz, G. E. (2004). Measuring effects of music, noise, and healing energy using a seed germination bioassay. *The Journal of Alternative and Complementary Medicine, 10*(1), 113-122. https://doi.org/10.1089/107555304322849047

[149] Radin, D., Stone, J., Levine, E., Eskandarnejad, S., Schlitz, M., Kozak, L., Mandel, D., & Hayssen, G. (2008). Compassionate intention as a therapeutic intervention by partners of cancer patients: Effects of distant intention on the patients' autonomic nervous system. *EXPLORE, 4*(4), 235-243. https://doi.org/10.1016/j.explore.2008.04.002

[150] Radin, D., et al. "Compassionate Intention as a Therapeutic Intervention by Partners of Cancer Patients: Effects of Distant Intention on the Patients' Autonomic Nervous System." *Explore,* July-Aug. 2008.

[151] Down, W. L. S. (2020). *Intentions Can Be Met Through Focused Consciousness Alone; Evidence We Can Realize Our Goals by Interacting with Them as Waves in the Unified Field* (Doctoral dissertation, International Quantum University for Integrative Medicine).

[152] "The Rhine Research Center Proves PK Is Real with Edd Edwards." *EddEdwards.com*, https://web.archive.org/web/20200928012326/ https://eddedwards.com/the-rhine-research-center-proves-pk-is-real-with-edd-edwards/. Accessed 3 Oct. 2024.

[153] Tips, J. (2010). *The Healing Power Within: The Story of Natural Healing and Cellular Energy*. Apple-A-Day Press.

[154] Melse-Boonstra A. Bioavailability of Micronutrients From Nutrient-Dense Whole Foods: Zooming in on Dairy, Vegetables, and Fruits. Front Nutr. 2020 Jul 24;7:101. doi: 10.3389/fnut.2020.00101. PMID: 32793622; PMCID: PMC7393990.

[155] Kirschvink JL, Kobayashi-Kirschvink A, Woodford BJ. Magnetite biomineralization in the human brain. Proc Natl Acad Sci U S A. 1992 Aug 15;89(16):7683-7. doi: 10.1073/pnas.89.16.7683. PMID: 1502184; PMCID: PMC49775.

[156] Costa, José. "Oncogenic viruses." Encyclopedia Britannica, 12 Sep. 2024, https://www.britannica.com/science/cancer-disease/Cancer-causing-agents#ref750271:~:text=A%20large%20number,cancer%20to%20develop. Accessed 13 September 2024.

[157] Irigaray, P., Newby, J. A., Clapp, R., Hardell, L., Howard, V., Montagnier, L., Epstein, S., & Belpomme, D. (2007). Lifestyle-related factors and environmental agents causing cancer: An overview. *Biomedicine & Pharmacotherapy, 61*(10), 640-658. https://doi.org/10.1016/j.biopha.2007.10.006

[158] Ito, M., Masuda, N., Shinomiya, K., Endo, K., & Ito, K. (2013). Systematic analysis of neural projections reveals clonal composition of the Drosophila brain. *Current Biology, 23*(8), 644-655. https://doi.org/10.1016/j.cub.2013.03.015

[159] Gerber, R. (2001). *Vibrational medicine: The #1 handbook of subtle-energy therapies* (3rd ed.). Bear & Company

[160] McFadden, Johnjoe. *Johnjoe McFadden Official Website*, https://johnjoemcfadden.co.uk.

[161] "Professor Jim Al-Khalili CBE FRS HonFREng HonFInstP HonFIET." *University of Surrey,* https://www.surrey.ac.uk/people/jim-al-khalili.

[162] Bird, R. P., & Eskin, N. A. M. (2021). The emerging role of phosphorus in human health. *In Advances in Food and Nutrition Research* (Vol. 96, pp. 27-88). Academic Press. https://doi.org/10.1016/bs.afnr.2021.02.001

[163] Fazzino, Tera L.; Rohde, Kaitlyn; Sullivan, Debra K. (2019-11-01). "Hyper-palatable foods: Development of a quantitative definition and application to the US Food System Database." Obesity. 27 (11): 1761–1768. doi:10.1002/oby.22639

[164] Kessler, D. A. (2010). *The end of overeating: Taking control of the insatiable American appetite.* Rodale Books.

[165] "The Story of the Mahatma's Experiments with Food." *Comprehensive Website on the Life and Works of Mahatma Gandhi,* https://www.mkgandhi.org/articles/mahatmas-experiements-with-food.php.

[166] "Eating the Past: Henry Ford's Soy Obsession." *Utah Public Radio,* 1 Apr. 2024, https://www.upr.org/show/eating-the-past/2024-04-01/eating-the-past-henry-fords-soy-obsession.

[167] Benor, D. J. (2004). *Consciousness, bioenergy and healing: Self-healing and energy medicine for the 21st century* (Vol. 2). Wholistic Healing Publications.

[168] Senior, Winston B. (2003-11-08). "Robert Murray Ricketts." British Dental Journal. 195 (9): 545. doi:10.1038/sj.bdj.4810673. ISSN 0007-0610. S2CID 35733954

[169] DiGeronimo, T. F., & Clement, B. R. (1998). *Living Foods for Optimum Health: Staying Healthy in an Unhealthy World.* Harmony.

[170] "David Williams." *Linus Pauling Institute,* Oregon State University, https://lpi.oregonstate.edu/faculty-staff/david-williams.

[171] "Dr. Konstantin Korotkov and the Study of the Human Energy Light System." *Biovie,* https://www.biovie.fr/en/blog/dr-konstantin-korotkov-and-the-study-of-the-human-energy-light-system-n43.

[172] Bista, S., & Bhargav, H. (2020). *Electro-photonic imaging: Measure your subtle energy level.*

[173] Korotkov, K. (2014). *Energy Fields Electrophotonic Analysis in Humans and Nature* (2nd ed.). [Translated from Russian by the author; Edited by B. Williams & L. Rabe].

[174] Kant, A. K., Schatzkin, A., Graubard, B. I., & Schairer, C. (2000). A prospective study of diet quality and mortality in women. *Jama,* 283(16), 2109-2115.

[175] "Bernard Grad." *PSI Encyclopedia,* Society for Psychical Research, https://psi-encyclopedia.spr.ac.uk/articles/bernard-grad.

[176] Grad, B. (1972). *Science investigates laying on of hands.* In *The Mind in Search of Itself* (Conference proceedings). Mind Science Foundation and Silva International, Washington, D.C. Retrieved from http://www.silvamentaldynamicscenter.com/PDF/hands.pdf

[177] Gerber, Richard. *Vibrational Medicine: The #1 Handbook of Subtle-Energy Therapies.*

[178] "Sister Justa Smith, Chairwoman of Chemistry at Rosary Hill, Dies." *The Buffalo News,* https://buffalonews.com/news/sister-justa-smith-chairwoman-of-chemistry-at-rosary-hill-dies/article_c05c8c94-1229-58e3-ae0e-358538cb07a7.html.

[179] Smith, M. J. (1972). Paranormal effects on enzyme activity. *Human Dimensions.*

[180] Gerber, R. (2001). *A practical guide to vibrational medicine: Energy healing and spiritual transformation.* HarperOne.

[181] "Dolores (Dee) Krieger (1921-2019)." *Nursology,* 1 Oct. 2019, https://nursology.net/2019/10/01/dolores-dee-krieger-1921-2019/

[182] Krieger, D. "Healing by the Laying-On of Hands as a Facilitator of Bioenergetic Change: The Response of In-Vivo Hemoglobin." *International Journal of Psychoenergetic Systems,* vol. 1, 1976, p. 121.

[183] Krieger, D. "Therapeutic Touch: The Imprimatur of Nursing." *American Journal of Nursing,* vol. 75, 1975, pp. 784-787.

[184] Krieger, Dolores. *Therapeutic Touch.* Simon and Schuster, 1979.

[185] Burgess JE, Gorton KL, Lasiter S, Patel SE. The Nurses' Perception of Expressive Touch: An Integrative Review. J Caring Sci. 2023 Feb 7;12(1):4-13. doi: 10.34172/jcs.2023.31903. PMID: 37124409; PMCID: PMC10131170.

[186] Benor, D. J. (2004). *Consciousness, bioenergy and healing: Self healing and energy medicine for the 21st century.* Wholistic Healing Publications.

[187] https://hameroff.arizona.edu/research-overview/orch-or

[188] Kalra, A. P., & Scholes, G. D., et al. (2023). Electronic energy migration in microtubules. *ACS Central Science, 9*(3). https://doi.org/10.1021/acscentsci.2c01114

[189] Li, N., Lu, D., Yang, L., Tao, H., Xu, Y., Wang, C., Fu, L., Liu, H., Chummum, Y., & Zhang, S. (2018). Nuclear spin attenuates the anesthetic potency of xenon isotopes in mice: Implications for the mechanisms of anesthesia and consciousness. *Anesthesiology, 129*(2), 271-277.

[190] Kosik, K. S. (2024). Why brain organoids are not conscious yet. *Patterns, 5*(8), 101011.

[191] "Research: Human Brain Organogenesis." *Muotri Lab,* University of California San Diego, https://pediatrics.ucsd.edu/research/faculty-labs/muotri-lab/index.html.

[192] *New Scientist.* https://www.newscientist.com/

[193] Margo, C. E. (1999). The placebo effect. *Survey of Ophthalmology, 44*(1), 31-44. https://doi.org/10.1016/S0039-6257(99)00060-0

[194] McCallum, R. W., & Berkowitz, D. M. (1976). Placebo effect in the treatment of duodenal ulcer. *Gastroenterology, 71*(5), 640-643.

[195] Moayyedi, P., & Delaney, B. (2002). The placebo effect in the treatment of peptic ulcer disease: A randomized controlled trial. *Alimentary Pharmacology & Therapeutics, 16*(5), 703-711. https://doi.org/10.1046/j.1365-2036.2002.01224.x

[196] Moseley, J. B., O'Malley, K., Petersen, N. J., Menke, T. J., Brody, B. A., Kuykendall, D. H., Hollingsworth, J. C., Ashton, C. M., & Wray, N. P. (2002). A controlled trial of arthroscopic surgery for osteoarthritis of the knee. *New England Journal of Medicine, 347*(2), 81-88. https://doi.org/10.1056/NEJMoa013259

[197] Fielding, J. W. L., Fagg, S. L., Jones, B. G., Ellis, D., Hockey, M. S., Minawa, A., Brookes, V. S., Craven, J. L., Mason, M. C., Timothy, A., Waterhouse, J. A. H., & Wrigley, P. F. M. (1983). An interim report of a prospective, randomized, controlled study of adjuvant chemotherapy in operable gastric cancer: British stomach cancer group. *World Journal of Surgery, 7*(3), 396-407. https://doi.org/10.1007/BF01658089

[198] Zajicek, Gershom. *ResearchGate,* https://www.researchgate.net/profile/Gershom-Zajicek.

[199] Zajicek G, "The placebo effect is the healing force of nature," The Cancer Journal 1995 Mar-Apr; 8(2).

[200] Nitzan, U., & Lichtenberg, P. (2004). Questionnaire survey on use of placebo. *BMJ,* 329(7472), 944. https://doi.org/10.1136/bmj.38236.646678.55

[201] Thomas, Kelly B. "General Practice Consultations: Is There Any Point in Being Positive?" *British Medical Journal (Clinical Research Edition),* vol. 294, no. 6581, 1987, pp. 1200-1202.

[202] "Dr. Herbert Benson." *Benson-Henry Institute for Mind Body Medicine,* https://bensonhenryinstitute.org/about-us-dr-herbert-benson/.

[203] Benson, H., & Stark, M. (1997). *Timeless healing.* Scribner.

[204] "Allen D. Roses." *American Neurological Association,* https://myana.org/allen-d-roses.

[205] https://www.the-independent.com/news/science/glaxo-chief-our-drugs-do-not-work-on-most-patients-5508670.html

[206] Kirsch, I., Deacon, B. J., Huedo-Medina, T. B., Scoboria, A., Moore, T. J., & Johnson, B. T. (2008). Initial severity and antidepressant benefits: A meta-analysis of data submitted to the Food and Drug Administration. *PLOS Medicine, 5*(2), e45. https://doi.org/10.1371/journal.pmed.0050045

[207] Madden, K. S., Felten, S. Y., Felten, D. L., Hardy, C. A., & Livnat, S. (1989). Sympathetic neural modulation of the immune system: I. Depression of T cell immunity in vivo and in vitro following chemical sympathectomy. *Brain, Behavior, and Immunity, 3*(1), 72-89. https://doi.org/10.1016/S0039-6257(99)00060-0

[208] Dispenza, J. (2014). *You are the placebo: Making your mind matter.* Hay House Inc.

[209] "Hippocrates Comprehensive Cancer Wellness Program." *Hippocrates Wellness,* https://hippocrateswellness.org/health-challenges/comprehensive-cancer-wellness-program.

[210] Lesniak, K. T. "The effect of intercessory prayer on wound healing in nonhuman primates." Alternative Therapies in Health & Medicine 12, no. 6 (November-December 2006): 42-48.

[211] Evans, H. (2010). Sliders: The Enigma of Streetlight Interference. United States: Anomalist Books.

[212] *Weird or What?* (2011, November 7). *Medical Mysteries* (Season 2, Episode 8) [TV series episode]. In W. Shatner (Host), Syfy. https://m.imdb.com/title/tt2096314/?ref_=ext_shr_lnk

[213] "Prof. Dr. Stuart Gilder." *Department of Earth and Environmental Sciences, Geophysics, Ludwig-Maximilians-Universität (LMU) München,* https://www.geophysik.uni-muenchen.de/en/Members/gilder. Accessed 3 Oct. 2024.

[214] Servick, K. (2019, March 18). Humans—like other animals—may sense Earth's magnetic field: But does this subconscious sense help us find our way? Science. https://www.science.org/content/article/humans-other-animals-may-sense-earth-s-magnetic-field

[215] Linton, O. (2006). *Ulrich Henschke. Journal of the American College of Radiology, 3*(8), 639. https://doi.org/10.1016/j.jacr.2006.03.016

[216] Proud, L. (2014). *Strange electromagnetic dimensions: The science of the unexplainable.* Weiser.

[217] "Most Lightning Strikes Survived." *Guinness World Records,* https://www.guinnessworldrecords.com/world-records/most-lightning-strikes-survived. Accessed 3 Oct. 2024.

[218] Dubey, R. (2022). *Impact of toxic anger on health (mind, body, soul). NeuroQuantology, 20*(14), 1-5.

[219] Weiss, Cynthia. "Mayo Clinic Q and A: Reducing Stress in the New Year." *Mayo Clinic News Network,* 2 Jan. 2023, https://newsnetwork.mayoclinic.org/discussion/mayo-clinic-q-and-a-reducing-stress-in-the-new-year/.

[220] Esch, T., & Stefano, G. B. (2011). The neurobiological link between compassion and love. *Medical science monitor : international medical journal of experimental and clinical research, 17*(3), RA65–RA75. https://doi.org/10.12659/msm.881441

[221] Vlachakis, C., Dragoumani, K., Raftopoulou, S., Mantaiou, M., Papageorgiou, L., Champeris Tsaniras, S., Megalooikonomou, V., & Vlachakis, D. (2018). Human emotions on the onset of cardiovascular and small vessel related diseases. *In Vivo, 32*(4), 859-870. https://doi.org/10.21873/invivo.11320

[222] Colletti, M. (2003). *An exploratory study of the relationships among depressive symptomatology, cellular immune function, and health status in HIV-infected men.* Rush University, College of Nursing

[223] Zhao, Z. (2022, January). The influence of loving-kindness meditation on mental health—a systematic review. In 2021 *International Conference on Social Development and Media Communication* (SDMC 2021) (pp. 957-961). Atlantis Press.

[224] Garrison, Kathleen A., et al. "BOLD Signal and Functional Connectivity Associated with Loving Kindness Meditation." *Brain and Behavior,* vol. 4, no. 3, 2014, pp. 337-347. https://doi.org/10.1002/brb3.219.

[225] Arias, Albert J., et al. "Systematic Review of the Efficacy of Meditation Techniques as Treatments for Medical Illness." *Journal of Alternative and Complementary Medicine,* vol. 12, no. 8, 11 Oct. 2006, https://doi.org/10.1089/acm.2006.12.817.

[226] Carson, James W., et al. "Loving-Kindness Meditation for Chronic Low Back Pain: Results From a Pilot Trial." *Journal of Holistic Nursing,* vol. 23, no. 3, Sept. 2005, pp. 287-304, https://doi.org/10.1177/0898010105277651.

[227] Tonelli, Makenzie E., and Amy B. Wachholtz. "Meditation-Based Treatment Yielding Immediate Relief for Meditation-Naïve Migraineurs." *Pain Management Nursing,* vol. 15, no. 1, Mar. 2014, pp. 36-40, https://doi.org/10.1016/j.pmn.2012.04.002.

[228] Kemper, Kathi J., et al. "Loving-Kindness Meditation's Effects on Nitric Oxide and Perceived Well-Being: A Pilot Study in Experienced and Inexperienced Meditators." *Explore,* vol. 11, no. 1, Jan.-Feb. 2015, pp. 32-39, https://doi.org/10.1016/j.explore.2014.10.002.

[229] "Larry Dossey MD." *DosseyDossey.com,* https://www.dosseydossey.com/larry-dossey-md.

[230] Dossey, L. (2013). *One mind: How our individual mind is part of a greater consciousness and why it matters.* Hay House Inc.

[231] Dossey, L. (1995). *Healing words: The power of prayer and the practice of medicine.* HarperOne.

[232] Dossey, L. (2003). *Healing beyond the body: Medicine and the infinite reach of the mind.* Shambhala.

[233] "Fred Luskin." *Greater Good Science Center,* University of California, Berkeley, https://greatergood.berkeley.edu/profile/fred_luskin.

[234] Luskin, Frederic. "The Art of Forgiveness." *Stanford Medicine: Surviving Cancer,* https://med.stanford.edu/survivingcancer/coping-with-cancer/cancer-and-forgiveness.html.

[235] Luskin, F. (2003). *Forgive for good: A proven prescription for health and happiness.* HarperOne.

[236] Michaud, Ellen. "How to Forgive Yourself." *Prevention,* updated 22 Mar. 2022, https://www.prevention.com/life/g20512857/how-to-forgive-yourself-no-matter-what/.

237 Lawler-Row, Kathleen A., et al. "Forgiveness, Physiological Reactivity and Health: The Role of Anger." *International Journal of Psychophysiology,* vol. 68, no. 1, Apr. 2008, pp. 51-58, https://doi.org/10.1016/j.ijpsycho.2008.01.001.

238 Friedberg, Jennifer P., Sonia Suchday, and Danielle V. Shelov. "The Impact of Forgiveness on Cardiovascular Reactivity and Recovery." *International Journal of Psychophysiology,* vol. 65, no. 2, Aug. 2007, pp. 87-94, https://doi.org/10.1016/j.ijpsycho.2007.03.006.

239 Lawler, Kathleen A., et al. "The Unique Effects of Forgiveness on Health: An Exploration of Pathways." *Journal of Behavioral Medicine,* vol. 28, Apr. 2005, pp. 157-167, https://doi.org/10.1007/s10865-005-3665-2.

240 Carson, James W., et al. "Forgiveness and Chronic Low Back Pain: A Preliminary Study Examining the Relationship of Forgiveness to Pain, Anger, and Psychological Distress." *The Journal of Pain,* vol. 6, no. 2, Feb. 2005, pp. 84-91, https://doi.org/10.1016/j.jpain.2004.10.012.

241 Emmons, R. A., & McCullough, M. E. (2003). Counting blessings versus burdens: An experimental investigation of gratitude and subjective well-being in daily life. Journal of Personality and Social Psychology, 84(2), 377-389. https://doi.org/10.1037/0022-3514.84.2.377

242 "Robert Emmons, Professor Emeritus." *Department of Psychology, University of California, Davis,* https://psychology.ucdavis.edu/people/robert-emmons.

243 Emmons, Robert A., and Michael E. McCullough. "Counting Blessings Versus Burdens: An Experimental Investigation of Gratitude and Subjective Well-Being in Daily Life." *Journal of Personality and Social Psychology,* vol. 84, no. 2, 2003, pp. 377-389, https://psycnet.apa.org/buy/2003-01140-012.

244 Rein, G., & McCraty, R. (1993, June). Modulation of DNA by coherent heart frequencies. In *Proceedings of the Third Annual Conference of the International Society for the Study of Subtle Energy and Energy Medicine* (pp. 58-62).

245 Rein, G., & McCraty, R. (1993). Local and nonlocal effects of coherent heart frequencies on conformational changes of DNA. In *Proc. Joint USPA/IAPR Psychotronics Conf., Milwaukee, WI.*

246 "Cyberscan Professional Biofeedback Device." *CyberBioFeedbackScans.com,* http://www.cyberbiofeedbackscans.com/cyber-scan/

247 "What Is It?" *Bio-Well,* https://www.bio-well.com/. Accessed 3 Oct. 2024.

248 "Research." *Valarie V. Hunt,* http://valerievhunt.com/ VALERIEVHUNT.COM/Valerie_Hunt_Research.html

249 **Bernardi, L., Porta, C., & Sleight, P. (2006).** Cardiovascular, cerebrovascular, and respiratory changes induced by different types of music in musicians and non-musicians: The importance of silence. Heart, 92(4), 445-452. https://doi.org/10.1136/hrt.2005.064600

250 Akimoto, K., Hu, A., Yamaguchi, T., & Kobayashi, H. (2018). Effect of 528 Hz music on the endocrine system and autonomic nervous system. *Health, 10*(09), 1159.

251 Meymandi A. (2009). Music, medicine, healing, and the genome project. *Psychiatry (Edgmont (Pa. : Township)), 6*(9), 43–45.

252 International Organization for Standardization. (1975). *ISO 16:1975(en) Acoustics — Standard tuning frequency (Standard musical pitch).* Retrieved September 16, 2024, from https://www.iso.org/obp/ui/#iso:std:iso:16:ed-1:v1:en

253 Ohno, S., & Ohno, M. (1986). The all pervasive principle of repetitious recurrence governs not only coding sequence construction but also human endeavor in musical composition. *Immunogenetics, 24,* 71-78.

254 Jenny, H. (1967). *Cymatics: A study of wave phenomena & vibration.* Macromedia.

255 MAHER-LOUGHNAN, G. P., MASON, A. A., MACDONALD, N., & FRY, L. (1962). Controlled trial of hypnosis in the symptomatic treatment of asthma. *British medical journal, 2*(5301), 371–376. https://doi.org/10.1136/bmj.2.5301.371

256 Williams, J. E. (1974). Stimulation of breast growth by hypnosis. *The Journal of Sex Research, 10*(4), 316–326. https://doi.org/10.1080/00224497409550865

257 Smith, A. P. (1998). *The power of thought to heal: An ontology of personal faith.* The Claremont Graduate University.

258 Nelson, Valerie J. "O. Carl Simonton Dies at 66; Oncologist Pioneered Mind-Body Connection to Fight Cancer." *Los Angeles Times,* 29 Sept. 2014, https://www.latimes.com/nation/la-me-carl-simonton3-2009jul03-story.html. Accessed 3 Oct. 2024.

[259] Antonelli, M.; Donelli, D.; Gurgoglione, F.L.; Lazzeroni, D.; Halasz, G.; Niccoli, G. Effects of Static Meditation Practice on Blood Lipid Levels: A Systematic Review and Meta-Analysis. *Healthcare* **2024**, *12*, 655. https://doi.org/10.3390/healthcare12060655

[260] Varma, Pooja, and Waheeda Khan. "Efficacy of Yoga and Meditation in Managing Hassles and Anxiety Among Angina Pectoris Patients." *Indian Journal of Community Psychology,* vol. 14, no. 1, 2018.

[261] Ko, D. (2005). Qigong for cancer: self-healing practice. *Townsend Letter for Doctors and Patients,* https://link.gale.com/apps/doc/A133803091/AONE?u=anon~957a95e5&sid=googleScholar&xid=c7d81d8e

[262] Federation of American Societies for Experimental Biology. (2007, April 25). Sea Squirt, Heal Thyself: Scientists Make Major Breakthrough In Regenerative Medicine. *ScienceDaily.* Retrieved September 16, 2024 from www.sciencedaily.com/releases/2007/04/070424093740.htm

[263] Witt C, Brinkhaus B, Jena S, et al. Acupuncture in patients with osteoarthritis of the knee: a randomised trial. *Lancet.* 2005;366(9480):136-143. doi:10.1016/S0140-6736(05)66871-7

[264] Martin DP, Sletten CD, Williams BA, Berger IH. Improvement in fibromyalgia symptoms with acupuncture: results of a randomized controlled trial. *Mayo Clin Proc.* 2006;81(6):749-757. doi:10.4065/81.6.749

[265] Emmons SL, Otto L. Acupuncture for overactive bladder: a randomized controlled trial. *Obstet Gynecol.* 2005;106(1):138-143. doi:10.1097/01.AOG.0000163258.57895.ec

[266] Lewith, G. T., White, P. J., & Pariente, J. (2005). Investigating acupuncture using brain imaging techniques: The current state of play. *Evidence-Based Complementary and Alternative Medicine,* 2(3), 315-319. https://doi.org/10.1093/ecam/neh110

[267] Huang, W., et al. "Characterizing Acupuncture Stimuli Using Brain Imaging with fMRI—A Systematic Review of the Literature." *European Journal of Integrative Medicine,* vol. 2, no. 4, 2010, p.209, https://doi.org/10.1016/j.eujim.2010.09.078.

[268] Wu, Chunxiao, et al. "Correlation Between the Effects of Acupuncture at Taichong (LR3) and Functional Brain Areas: A Resting-State Functional Magnetic Resonance Imaging Study Using True Versus Sham Acupuncture." *Evidence-Based Complementary and Alternative Medicine,* 22 May 2014, https://doi.org/10.1155/2014/729091.

[269] Benor DJ. *Consciousness, Bioenergy, and Healing: Self-Healing and Energy Medicine for the 21st Century.* Wholistic Healing Publications; 2004:181.

[270] Oschman, James. *Researcher Profile. ResearchGate,* https://www.researchgate.net/profile/James-Oschman.

[271] Lim, T. K., Ma, Y., Berger, F., & Litscher, G. (2018). Acupuncture and Neural Mechanism in the Management of Low Back Pain- An Update. *Medicines (Basel, Switzerland), 5*(3), 63. https://doi.org/10.3390/medicines5030063

[272] Deng, H., & Shen, X. (2013). The mechanism of moxibustion: ancient theory and modern research. *Evidence-Based Complementary and Alternative Medicine, 2013*(1), 379291.

[273] Britannica, The Editors of Encyclopaedia. "Richard Leakey." Encyclopedia Britannica, 21 Mar. 2024, https://www.britannica.com/biography/Richard-Leakey. Accessed 18 September 2024.

[274] Leakey, R. E. F., & Lewin, R. (1977). Origins: What new discoveries reveal about the emergence of our species and its possible future.

[275] Harman, D. (1992). Free radical theory of aging. *Mutation Research/DNAging, 275*(3-6), 257-266.

[276] Harman, D. (2009). Origin and evolution of the free radical theory of aging: A brief personal history, 1954–2009. *Biogerontology, 10*(6), 773–781. https://doi.org/10.1007/s10522-009-9234-2

[277] "Emotional Freedom Technique: Research Supports Benefits of Tapping for Mental Health." *Purdue University,* 2023, https://www.purdue.edu/newsroom/purduetoday/2023/Q3/emotional-freedom-technique-research-supports-benefits-of-tapping-for-mental-health/

[278] "Dr. Roger Callahan (8th May 1925 – 4th November 2013)." *The Guild of Energists,* https://goe.ac/dr_roger_callahan.htm. Accessed 3 Oct. 2024.

[279] Callahan, R. (2023, June 8). *Alternatives spawned from Thought Field Therapy.* Roger Callahan's Official Website. Retrieved September 18, 2024, from https://web.archive.org/web/20230608085304/http://www.rogercallahan.com/callahan.php#:~:text=Alternatives%20Spawned%20From,Training%20in%201999

[280] Feinstein D. Energy psychology: A review of the preliminary evidence. *Psychotherapy (Chic).* 2008;45(2):199-213. doi:10.1037/0033-3204.45.2.199

[281] Ortner, Nick. *The tapping solution for pain relief: A step-by-step guide to reducing and eliminating chronic pain.* Hay House, 2015.

[282] Stapleton, P., et al. "A Randomized Clinical Trial of a Meridian-Based Intervention for Food Cravings with Six-Month Follow-Up." *Behaviour Change,* 2011

[283] Stapleton, P., et al. "Clinical Benefits of Emotional Freedom Techniques on Food Cravings at 12-Months Follow-Up: A Randomized Controlled Trial." *Energy Psychology,* Mar. 2012

[284] Stapleton P, Roos T, Mackintosh G, Sparenburg E, Sabot D, Carter B. Online Delivery of Emotional Freedom Techniques in the Treatment of Food Cravings and Weight Management: A Randomised Controlled Trial. *OBM Integrative and Complementary Medicine* **2019**; 4(4): 065; doi:10.21926/obm.icm.1904065.

[285] Church, D. "Reductions in Pain, Depression, and Anxiety Symptoms After PTSD Remediation in Veterans." *Explore,* vol. 10, no. 3, May-June 2014, pp. 162-169

[286] Babamahmoodi, A., et al. "Emotional Freedom Technique (EFT) Effects on Psychoimmunological Factors of Chemically Pulmonary Injured Veterans." *Iran Journal of Allergy, Asthma, and Immunology,* vol. 14, no. 1, Feb. 2015, pp. 37-47.

[287] Salas, M. M., et al. "The Immediate Effect of a Brief Energy Psychology Intervention (Emotional Freedom Techniques) on Specific Phobias: A Pilot Study." *Explore,* vol. 7, no. 3, May-June 2011, pp. 155-161

[288] Clement, B. R., & Clement, A. M. (2023). *Self healing diet: A scientifically supported, life-awakening guide revealing the impact our lifestyle choices have on our health, longevity, and environment.* Hippocrates Publications.

[289] Feinstein, D. "Energy Psychology: A Review of the Preliminary Evidence." *Psychotherapy,* June 2008.

[290] Feinstein, D. "The Case of Energy Psychology." *Psychotherapy Networker,* 2010

[291] Ruden, R. A. (2005). A Neurological Basis for the Observed Peripheral Sensory Modulation of Emotional Responses. Traumatology, 11(3), 145-158. https://doi.org/10.1177/153476560501100301

[292] Ruden, Ronald A. "Why Tapping Works - A Sense for Healing: The Neurobiological Basis of Peripheral Sensory Stimulation for Modulation of Emotional Response." *Healing the Mind,* Mar. 2005, https://web.archive.org/web/20150215172255/www.healingthemind.net/html/Why_tapping_works.html. Accessed 3 Oct. 2024.

[293] Andrade, J., & Feinstein, D. (2003). Preliminary report of the first large scale study of energy psychology. *Energy Psychology Interactive: An Integrated Book and CD Program for Learning the Fundamentals of Energy Psychology.*

[294] Andrade, J., and David Feinstein. "Preliminary Report of the First Large-Scale Study of Energy Psychology with Brain Scans." *EFT Research Paper,* Republished 2 Mar. 2015, https://www.efttappingtraining.com/eft-research-paper/preliminary-report-of-the-first-large-scale-study-of-energy-psychology-with-brain-scans/. Accessed 3 Oct. 2024.

[295] Williamson TK, Rodriguez HC, Gonzaba A, Poddar N, Norwood SM, Gupta A. H-Wave® Device Stimulation: A Critical Review. *Journal of Personalized Medicine.* 2021; 11(11):1134. https://doi.org/10.3390/jpm11111134

[296] Bianconi, E., Piovesan, A., Facchin, F., Beraudi, A., Casadei, R., Frabetti, F., ... & Canaider, S. (2013). An estimation of the number of cells in the human body. *Annals of Human Biology, 40*(6), 463-471. https://doi.org/10.3109/03014460.2013.807878

[297] de Oliveira, R. F., de Andrade Salgado, D. M. R., Trevelin, L. T., et al. (2015). Benefits of laser phototherapy on nerve repair. *Lasers in Medical Science, 30*(5), 1395–1406. https://doi.org/10.1007/s10103-014-1531-6

[298] Michael J. Marino, Amber Luong, William C. Yao, Martin J. Citardi; Nonpharmacological Relaxation Technology for Office-Based Rhinologic Procedures. *ORL* 16 April 2019; 81 (1): 48–54. https://doi.org/10.1159/000488323

[299] Hendryx, J., Kannan, A., Prashad, J., & Falk, K. (2022). Connecting the dots: Alterations in bioelectric activity at acupuncture Ting (Jing-Well) points following CV4 cranial manipulation. *Journal of Osteopathic Medicine.* https://doi.org/10.1515/jom-2022-0111

[300] Zyto Technologies. (2024). *Dr. Voll's Dermatron device and electrodermal screening.* Zyto Technologies. Retrieved September 18, 2024, from https://zyto.com/electrodermal-screening#:~:text=Dr.%20Voll%E2%80%99s%20Dermatron,each%20acupuncture%20point

[301] Char, J. (1980). *Electro-Acupuncture for Dentistry, Paperback.* Lulu.com.

[302] "Björn Nordenström Dies." *Microwave News,* 11 Jan. 2007, https://microwavenews.com/news-center/bj%C3%B6rn-nordenstr%C3%B6m-. Accessed 3 Oct. 2024.

[303] Nordenstrom, B. E. (1989). Electrochemical treatment of cancer. I: Variable response to anodic and cathodic fields. *American journal of clinical oncology,* 12(6), 530-536.

[304] Nordenström, B. E., & Nordenström, J. (2004). The paradigm of biologically closed electric circuits and its clinical applications. In *Bioelectromagnetic Medicine* (pp. 678-687). CRC Press.

[305] Nordenström, B., Ipavec, S., & Alfas, S. (1992). Interferences of electromagnetic field with biological matter. *International Journal of Environmental Studies, 42*(2–3), 157–167. https://doi.org/10.1080/00207239208710792

[306] "Dr. Beverly Brubik." *Brubik,* https://www.brubik.com/

[307] Rubik, B. (n.d.). *Measurement of the human biofield and other energetic instruments* (Chapter 20 of "Energetics and Spirituality" by Lyn Freeman). Foundation for Alternative and Integrative Medicine. Retrieved September 18, 2024, from www.faim.org/measurement-of-the-human-biofield-and-other-energetic-instruments

[308] Baloh, R.W. (2024). The Early Age of Electrotherapy. In: Brain Electricity. Springer, Cham. https://doi.org/10.1007/978-3-031-62994-5_2

[309] Wylie, L. (2024, September 11). *Wellness app revenue and usage statistics (2024).* Business of Apps. Retrieved September 18, 2024, from https://www.businessofapps.com/data/wellness-app-market/

[310] The Business Research Company. (2024, January). *Wearable blood pressure monitors global market report 2024*

[311] Manasa, B., Jois, S. N., & Prasad, K. N. (2020). Prana – The vital energy in different cultures: Review on knowledge and practice. *Journal of Natural Remedies, 20*(2), 55-63. https://doi.org/10.18311/jnr/2020/24487

[312] Pollack, G. H. (2013). The fourth phase of water. *Ebner and Sons Publishers: Seattle, WA, USA.*

[313] Dispenza, J. (2014). *You are the placebo: Making your mind matter* (p. 197). Hay House.

[314] Watson, J. D., & Crick, F. H. C. (1953). Molecular structure of nucleic acids: A structure for deoxyribose nucleic acid. Nature, 171(4356), 737-738. https://doi.org/10.1038/171737a0

[315] Levin, M., & Martyniuk, C. J. (2018). The bioelectric code: An ancient computational medium for dynamic control of growth and form. *Biosystems, 164,* 76-93.

[316] California State University Northridge. (n.d.). *Chief Seattle's letter to all.* Retrieved September 18, 2024, from https://www.csun.edu/~vcpsy00h/seattle.htm

[317] Padavic-Callaghan, K. (2024, September 7). Reality's comeback. *New Scientist, 263*(3507), 32-35. https://doi.org/10.1016/S0262-4079(24)01613-0

[318] Rugai, J., & Hamiliton-Ekeke, J. T. (2016). A Review of Digital Addiction: A Call for Safety Education. *Journal of Education and e-Learning Research, 3*(1), 17-22.

[319] Rossano, G. F., Martinez, C., Hedelind, M., Murphy, S., & Fuhlbrigge, T. A. (2013, August). Easy robot programming concepts: An industrial perspective. In *2013 IEEE international conference on automation science and engineering (CASE)* (pp. 1119-1126). IEEE.

[320] Britannica, T. Editors of Encyclopaedia (2024, May 27). Norman Vincent Peale. Encyclopedia Britannica. https://www.britannica.com/biography/Norman-Vincent-Peale

[321] Peale, N. V. (1952). *The power of positive thinking* (p. 9). Prentice Hall

HIPPOCRATES
WELLNESS

PIONEERS of LONGEVITY
SINCE 1956

ENLIGHTENED LITERATURE
FURTHER READING BY BRIAN R. CLEMENT PH.D., L.N.

Killer Fish
Brian R. Clement
PhD, NMD, LN

Living Foods for Optimum Health
Brian R. Clement
PhD, NMD, LN

Self-Healing Diet
Brian R. Clement
PhD, NMD, LN
Anne Maria Clement
PhD, NMD, LN

Live to 120
Elliot G. Levy M.D.
Brian R. Clement
PhD, NMD, LN

QUANTUM HUMAN
Brian R. Clement
PhD, NMD, LN

Discovering You in You
Brian R. Clement
PhD, NMD, LN
Katherine C Powell
Ed.D.

Sweet Disease
Brian R. Clement
PhD, NMD, LN

Belief: Integrity in Relationships
Brian R. Clement PhD, NMD, LN
Katherine Powell, Ed.D.

The Power of a Woman
Anne Maria Clement
PhD, NMD, LN
Katherine C. Powell
Ed.D.

Lifeforce
Brian R. Clement
PhD, NMD, LN

Killer Clothes
Brian R. Clement
PhD, NMD, LN
Anne Maria Clement
PhD, NMD, LN

Manopause
Brian R. Clement
PhD, NMD, LN

Poison Poultry
Brian R. Clement
PhD, NMD, LN

Healthful Cuisine
Anne Maria Clement
PhD, NMD, LN
Kelly Serbonich

Dairy Deception
Brian R. Clement
PhD, NMD, LN

Longevity: Enjoying Long Life without Limits
Brian R. Clement
PhD, NMD, LN

Health & Healing
Brian R. Clement
PhD, NMD, LN

7 Keys to Lifelong Sexual Vitality
Brian R. Clement
PhD, NMD, LN
Anne Maria Clement
PhD, NMD, LN

The 'Food is Medicine' Series
Brian R. Clement
PhD, NMD, LN

Scan the QR Code to visit the Hippocrates Store
or visit: store.hippocrateswellness.org/collections/books

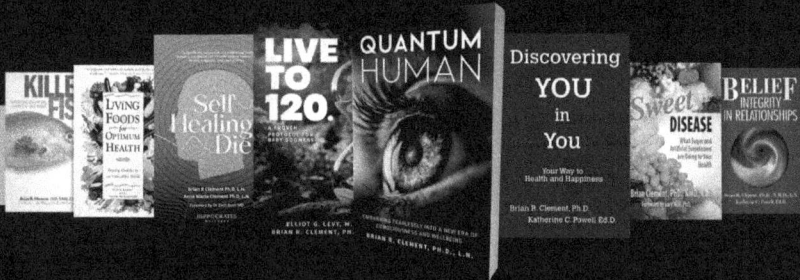

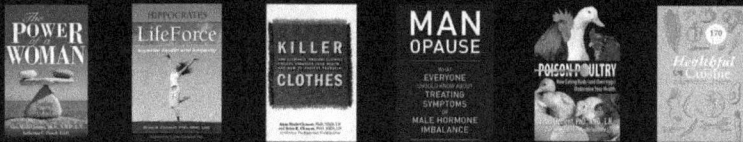

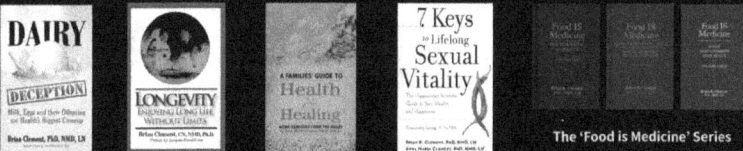

TRANSFORMATIVE PLANT-BASED RECIPES

QUANTUM
Cuisine

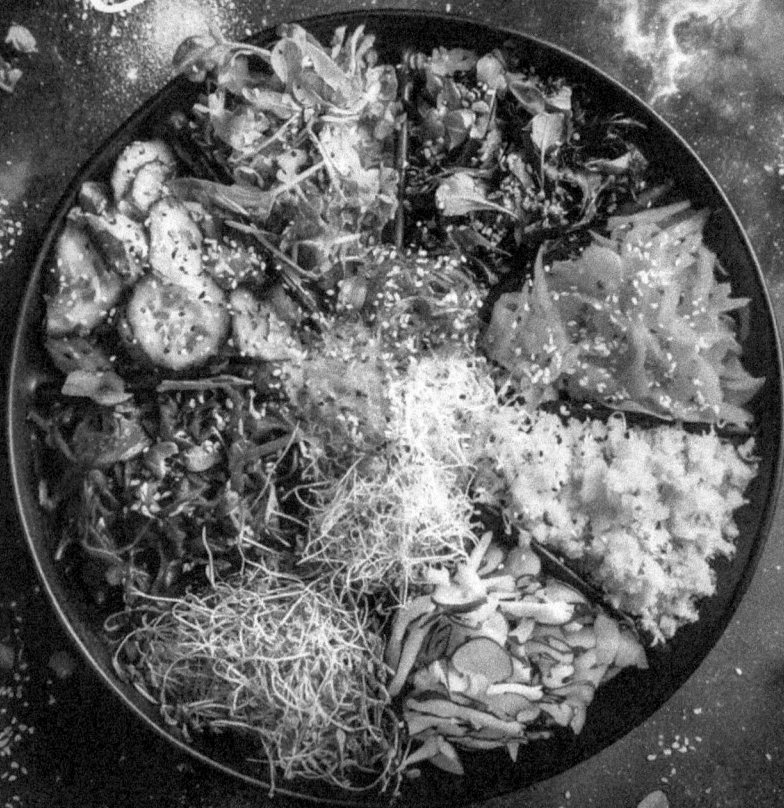

ANNA MARIA CLEMENT PH.D., L.N.
& EXECUTIVE CHEF KEN BLUE D.M.Q.

Powered by

HIPP♦CRATES
WELLNESS

PIONEERS *of* LONGEVITY
SINCE 1956

www.ingramcontent.com/pod-product-compliance
Lightning Source LLC
Chambersburg PA
CBHW050648270326
41927CB00012B/2919